Breast Cancer Q & A is like Cliffs Notes for cancer patients. At precisely the moment in time when you most need straight, clear answers, this book gives it to you without a lot of fluff or fuss. A fabulous resource!

—JENNIE NASH, author of *The Victoria's Secret Catalog Never Stops Coming and Other Lessons I Learned From Breast Cancer*

It is always refreshing to see a new book about breast cancer that provides something different and useful that has been lacking in the past. The question-and-answer format in this guide provides a well-organized and informative framework over a vast range of topics.

—DEBU TRIPATHY, M.D., University of Texas Southwestern Medical Center

This book clearly and concisely provides knowledge to those who seek to be informed . . . [on topics ranging] from diagnosis to reconstructive surgery.

—SHERRY STERLING, R.N., B.S., Sr. Research Nurse, M. D. Anderson Cancer Center

BREAST CANCER Q&A

. . . .

Insightful Answers to the 100 Most
Frequently Asked Questions

. . . .

Charyn Pfeuffer

AVERY
a member of Penguin Group (USA) Inc.
New York

a member of
Penguin Group (USA) Inc.
375 Hudson Street
New York, NY 10014
www.penguin.com

Library of Congress Cataloging-in-Publication Data

Breast cancer Q & A : insightful answers to the 100 most frequently
asked questions / Charyn Pfeuffer.
p.   cm.
Includes bibliographical references and index.
ISBN 1-58333-145-X (alk. paper)
1. Breast—Cancer—Popular works.   2. Breast—Cancer—Miscellanea.   I. Title: Breast
cancer Q and A.   II. Title: Breast cancer questions and answers.

RC280.B8B6877   2003   2003040409
616.99'449—dc21

Printed in the United States of America
1   3   5   7   9   10   8   6   4   2

Book design by Amanda Dewey

In memory of my mother,
Christine Ayn Pfeuffer

Acknowledgments

Sincere thanks go to:

Matthew Rowe, your unconditional love, support, and energy are a constant source of personal and professional inspiration. May our experiences be never ending.

My family: Dad, Pat, Carrie, David, and Ted, for proving that life's most difficult challenges sometimes prove to be our greatest blessings.

Carol Susan Roth, my literary agent, for recognizing this project's potential, for all of her developmental input and expertise, and for helping to bring this book to fruition with relentless fervor.

Laura Shepherd and Kristen Jennings, my editors at Avery/Penguin. Your guidance and enthusiasm has made the publishing process painless. Thank you to everyone else at Avery, including Amanda Dewey, designer extraordinaire, who had a talented hand in this project.

Lillie Shockney, a survivor of breast cancer, who's been there and back. Thank you for selflessly sharing your woman-to-woman wisdom, and for your assistance and invaluable feedback in reviewing this book from cover to cover.

Beverly Burns, for giving complementary medicine a voice in the world and for contributing her extensive expertise in reviewing this book.

Jennifer Jones, for contributing her time and artistic talent to this project.

To the women *living* with breast cancer, Carol Olby, Pat Moody, Diane Pecher, Stacey Sforza, Amy Spiegel, and Barbara McCoart, who so candidly offered their "if I'd only known" advice, laughter, tears, opinions, bitches, complaints, and experiences about breast cancer. I am in awe of your strength, and appreciative of your contributions.

The volunteers and staff of the Women's Cancer Resource Center, especially Diane Estrin, for selflessly giving their special gift of support, listening, and kindness to women with all types of cancer.

Marc Rand, who was there for everything. A decade later, your friendship is still an unwavering source of strength.

My friends, for your unconditional support, for checking in when I sometimes felt like I was checking out, and for tolerating countless last-minute cancellations when I couldn't stop writing. Thank you for truly understanding the personal importance of this project.

Tammy Dyson, for encouraging volunteerism and for being such a kindhearted individual. You helped bring me to where I am now, and I am thankful.

Joanne Bussiere, for not letting breast cancer or a brain tumor get the best of her, her gift of spontaneous giggling and for contributing her brilliant insights on life to this book.

Rachel Naomi Remen, whose words and wisdom have made me realize that it doesn't take much to make a difference in the world (or your own backyard).

Robert Young and Shawn Kresal. May Kristin's generous spirit and feisty attitude resonate in our daily lives. For the all-too-brief period that our lives intersected, she affected me profoundly. Thank you.

Contents

Foreword

All I want, I boldly said, is to keep you from dying, with my love: and the wasp sting was so deep, all my flesh was a crater to it.

—Joyce Carol Oates

It is ironic that I write this foreword as Mother's Day approaches. Every Mother's Day is bittersweet for me, and I think, too, for the author of this book, Charyn Pfeuffer. We both lost our mothers to cancer—Charyn when she was only 17. While her father worked, she assumed the responsibility of taking care of her 14-year-old sister and of her mother as she became increasingly ill. Her mother was misdiagnosed twice before lung cancer was confirmed. Immediately Charyn headed to the library to research anything she could find.

A great deal of information existed on lung cancer, but there was a limited amount on treatments for this disease and their side effects. There was also little patient support available to her. Charyn and her mother's questions were often ignored and dismissed. With no answers, Charyn decided to seek counseling in order to find answers and comfort for herself as well as for her mother. I once asked her how she knew to do all this, and at such a young age. She simply responded, "I just know when to ask for help." But, as I spoke with her, I realized that there was much more there.

I first met Charyn at the Women's Cancer Research Center's 2001 Swim-A-Mile for Women with Cancer fund-raising committee meeting. She volunteered to help recruit food donations. Her hand was always flying into the air, volunteering for other tasks! I knew she was volunteering in other parts of the Center's programs but this was the first time I actually connected with her. I can remember thinking how refreshing it was to work with someone so enthusiastic and dedicated to supporting the work of the Center. She still volunteers for the swim, but also comes in weekly to answer the Center's Information and Referral Helpline.

I recently had the fortune to run into her at the Information and Referral desk, and I asked her how she was doing. She replied with her usual smile that she "loves talking directly to the women and being able to help" and then she gives me a big hug! Charyn once described her mother as "a social butterfly that made everything happen in the family. . . . Mom had lots of energy." Well, guess what? You can see this energy emanating out of Charyn: she is indeed her mother's daughter.

When we talked about her wanting to write this book, I wondered why is she writing about breast and not lung cancer? The answer was not too far away. Charyn's eager tone changed when she spoke of not having any choices regarding her mother's treatment; of not knowing how to help; of trying to know, but not being able to find the right answers. She stopped and said without her usual smile, "I just want women to have a choice." Now, ten years after her mother's death, I can still see the anguish of a 17-year-old girl in her eyes. *Breast Cancer Q & A* is the answer to that torment. Anguish turned into action.

Jackie Winnow, the founder of the Women's Cancer Resource Center (WCRC), was a women's health activist, feminist, and lesbian when she was diagnosed with breast cancer in 1985. She writes "in the period between biopsy and diagnosis, my partner and I realized that we had to become cancer experts." Not unlike Charyn Pfeuffer, she was "hard hit by the reality that there was no place for me to go to empower myself. There was no central source of information where I could go to become an informed consumer of my own health care." So Jackie and her friend Carla Dalton began gathering information about how to survive and cope with her cancer. Soon, the word was out and women with cancer started calling, asking questions of the newly dubbed "cancer mavens." The Center has now grown into a multifaceted, nonprofit advocacy group and support and resource center for women with cancer. Out of one woman's necessity and drawn from the experience of many, the WCRC was conceived, as was this book.

This book embodies the collective voices of women with breast cancer, the earnest conscientiousness of that young girl, and the mission of the

Women's Cancer Resource Center. The WCRC helps women become empowered to make the decisions they need to make, to live the lives that they need to live. *Breast Cancer Q & A* does the same.

—Diane Estrin
Executive Director,
Women's Cancer Resource Center

Introduction

I never went to Europe," my mother sighed in a Percocet-induced state of delusion. (That comment was followed up with "And I can *never* have sex again," but I readily ignored that statement.) It was a Thursday night, exactly two weeks before my mother's 38-year-old body would surrender to metastatic lung cancer after a brief, half-year battle. At the time of her diagnosis, I was 17 years old, and cancer was a topic that had never, *ever* occurred to me. I grew up in a cookie-cutter Philadelphia suburb where, except for the occasional tragedy or accident, people just didn't die until they were good and ready. So you can imagine my shock and disbelief when I later found out that the best-case scenario was that my mother had three months to live. From the moment my family was handed the dreaded "C" diagnosis, I immediately embarked on an exasperating educational crash course in the world of cancer, health care, and medical experts.

My mother was first treated for what doctors thought was a blood clot in her right arm that resulted from overexertion. Although my mother was statuesque, she wasn't exactly Wonder Woman when it came to physical strength. If her right arm was ever overexerted, it was from lifting the cordless phone to her ear, obsessively vacuuming the house, schlepping shopping bags from Saks Fifth Avenue, or mixing five o'clock cocktails. I would later come to appreciate that she made up for her physical shortcomings in the emotional department.

The summer before my senior year in high school (1990), my mother, Christine Pfeuffer, spent in and out of the hospital. When she wasn't horizontal and hooked up to intravenous blood-thinning drips and taking smoke breaks with the nurses, she was taking a carefully timed, around-the-clock regimen of prescription drugs. Her condition was hardly improving, as her arm and neck swelled to unattractive proportions, and doctors kept fumbling for a possible diagnosis. One moment it was Hodgkin's disease, Lyme disease the next. My notion that doctors were all-knowing creatures (in the same realm as parents and teachers) slowly dissipated.

One hot-as-hell August day, when she was in the midst of a week-long inpatient stint at the hospital, her throat started constricting and she physically turned blue. Doctors were at a loss for what to do, and she was transported via helicopter to the intensive care unit of another Philadelphia-area hospital. When I arrived at the latest and greatest hospital, during the designated family-members-only visiting hours, and saw her semiconscious body, I realized the uncertainty and seriousness of her condition. I didn't know *what* was wrong with her, but for the first time, I knew that she could die.

A CT scan later, a suspicious mass was discovered. The mass was aspirated, and the fluid was sent out for a cell count and cytology evaluation. Cytology came back with Class IV cells, raising suspicions among the doctors of adenocarcinoma. A few days later, my mother's ever-changing condition had a name: non–small cell lung carcinoma. The doctors also made an alarming discovery: a tumor existed on the very first CT scan, which had been taken in June. The report accompanying the original CT scan said in the very last paragraph (on the fourth page) that the underlying problem was cancer. Two months later, it was the first we'd heard of it.

The new doctors were surprised that the original hospital and throng of doctors had not mentioned cancer, and were now reluctant to confirm how long she had had the disease. We skeptically wondered if she'd been transferred to cover the initial hospital's mistake. Lesson learned: It's crucial for the patient or the patient's advocate to review all X rays and reports and not take the doctor's word as the absolute truth.

Pissed off, but grateful to know what we were working with, I immediately set about researching the diagnosis and treatment options. The doctors had given us disappointingly little information to go on: a few photocopied handouts, a short recommended reading list, and numbers for family therapists. The books we did consult required medical dictionaries to simply navigate, let alone fully comprehend. I was scared to death, and so was the rest of my family. My mother was *dying,* for Chrissakes. I felt helpless, left in the dark, and appointments and treatments were being scheduled too fast to keep up. Making decisions, let alone informed decisions, was damn near impossible. As I look back on my mother's medical records, I wince at her scrawled signatures on countless consent forms, knowing that she had little knowledge of the choices she was making.

Once my mother was stable enough to be cared for at home, she started seeing doctors at a top-notch, specialized cancer center on an outpatient basis. She was consulted about the possibility of chemotherapy and radiation and managed to receive about a month of radiation treatments. The radiation was brutal on her fragile body, and every night I soothed her burned skin with lotions, tickled her back, and brushed her hair. It was the least I could do, and these simple pleasures brought her much joy. But her condition rapidly deteriorated, and doctors ruled out the possibility of chemotherapy. It was clear that she wasn't going to survive with or without chemo, but the doctors snatched this opportunity for a last-ditch effort away. Life was moving faster than ever, and although the doctors and nurses tried to keep us up to date on her status, we always felt two steps behind.

My mother's quality of life became the most important issue. We knew she was going to die; she was given three months to live, *maximum.* Throughout the dying process, my mother claimed minimal pain, but after one look, you knew she wasn't a very skilled liar. Women are rarely given societal permission to express feelings of pain or distress, and my mother prided herself on being the dutiful housewife and my father's secretary. Many women with cancer experience feelings of intense guilt if they dare kvetch about any of the side effects, such as pain, menopausal symptoms, psychosexual effects, and so on. They are living with cancer, and how dare they complain about anything else when their strength and focus should be on conquering this disease? Sheesh.

Doctors were endlessly adding to my mother's medicinal artillery. The more scrips they wrote, the less I recognized the woman my mother had morphed into. Her connection with reality was long gone, and although I found much-needed moments of comic respite in her hallucinations and delusions, I would've given anything for things to be as they'd been before cancer.

Exactly one week before my mother died, she was checked into the chi-chi suburban Philadelphia inpatient cancer clinic. She'd been on a never-ending wait list, but somehow my father finagled her admittance. The evening before she passed away, my dear friend Marc and I made the 45-minute schlep to the hospital bearing irises. I left her spa-like room knowing that would be the last time I would see her breathing. Sure enough, the following morning as I was driving around avoiding school, I had a lingering, sick feeling around 10:30. Lynard Skynard's "Free Bird" came on the radio. I don't particularly like classic rock, but for some coincidental reason, "Free Bird" would come on the radio at pivotal times throughout my mother's sickness.

I knew in my gut that she had passed away, and I knew that nobody would be able to find me. Reluctantly, I made an appearance at school, and my instinct was confirmed by the vice principal—the last man I would ever hope to be consoled by. The moment that my suspicions were verified, I knew *exactly* what I was supposed to do. I had always considered my mother the ultimate taskmaster, queen of the to-do list—but during what should've been an emotional meltdown, I thought of how she always handled herself. I needed to maintain some semblance of sanity, put one foot in front of the other and try to get myself and the rest of my family through this.

Fast-forward a decade: my father married an amazing woman—a high school teacher and a wildly creative and insightful woman. I acquired two incredible stepbrothers in the process, and have grown considerably closer to my sister, Carrie. Yes, I still mourn the loss of my mother, but I have learned to rejoice in the positive things that life has dealt me as a result. Cancer makes you take a step back and reexamine your life and what you want it to mean. My mother's brave spirit, and her words, "I never went to Europe," have inspired me to live my life fully, kindly, spontaneously, and with purpose.

When I moved to San Francisco in 2000, I desperately wanted to give something back to my community. I'm a freelance journalist with a flexible schedule and a hunger for human interaction. As much as I love my 10-second daily commute to my trusty computer, giving dating advice to girlfriends via Instant Messenger isn't exactly what I had in mind in terms of a humanitarian contribution.

I found the Women's Cancer Resource Center (WCRC) in Berkeley, California, participated in an intense training program, and immediately began volunteering. At WCRC, I assist with the annual fund-raising event (Swim-A-Mile) and staff the Information and Referral Helpline once a week. Breast cancer is an issue that comes up far too frequently, and, as a woman, it's hard not to take notice. Calls from women with cancer, their friends, coworkers, employers, family members, and loved ones flood the Helpline, helping me to refine my listening skills. As a volunteer, I am able to provide these panic-stricken women with immediate information about support groups and services, traditional and complementary treatment options, and information on local physicians and other health care providers.

I think it's important for women to evaluate *all* of their treatment options, both conventional and complementary. Much of the information and opinions currently available are biased toward one method or another, and I hope to present many of the possibilities free of heavy medical jargon. Much of the research for this book was conducted at WCRC's extensive library. And since you won't find a Ph.D., M.D., or R.N. after my name, I've had the appropriate information reviewed by two women who are experts in their respective fields. The first, Lillie Shockney, is a breast cancer survivor and the director of education and outreach at the Johns Hopkins Breast Center. Second, Beverly Burns is a mother, practicing acupuncturist, and clinical director of the Charlotte Maxwell Complementary Clinic in Berkeley. I asked Diane Estrin to write the foreword, since my experiences at WCRC have far exceeded any expectations I may have had. I sincerely want women near and far to know about all of the wonderful services and comfort that WCRC provides. It has been sort of an extended family for me. And to return the support these groups have provided me, a percentage of the proceeds of this book will be donated to these incredible women's organizations.

Breast cancer is by far the most common cancer among women. This year, breast cancer will account for nearly one out of every three cancer diagnoses in women. The good news is that an estimated 2,167,000 women are *living* with breast cancer. These shocking statistics and my personal experiences with cancer, however, prompted me to write this book. If a woman hasn't been affected by breast cancer, she is at risk. Over 70 percent of breast cancers occur in women who have no identifiable risk factors other than age, and only 5 to 10 percent of breast cancers are linked to a family history of breast cancer.

Whether you're newly diagnosed, in the midst of treatment, picking up the pieces posttreatment, or facing a recurrence, coping with breast cancer can be a frightening journey. A diagnosis of cancer inevitably brings with it countless questions, and becoming an instant breast cancer authority can be overwhelming. Whatever your reaction may be, it is normal. Cry, get angry, feel fear, scream and shout, belt out some Aretha Franklin, or do whatever it is that you need to do. In this time of crisis, you must become your own advocate. I cannot emphasize enough the importance of patient empowerment. Whatever your questions or concerns, you should *never* hesitate to share them with your treatment team. You'll be faced with making difficult decisions that you may not feel comfortable making. That said, doing research on your own can make the dialogue with your treatment team much more productive. It is essential to remember that you have time to gather information, and then make decisions based on the facts and personal considerations (i.e., your lifestyle, emotional well-being, and philosophies)—not knee-jerk emotional responses. Remember:

This is your life and your breast.
You are an individual, not a statistic.
You have needs that are unique to you.
Information is a valuable tool.

You have every right to be involved and in control
of your medical care and decisions.
Questioning authority, respectfully, is often difficult and fraught
with self-doubt. Doing so is often necessary and productive.
One should do so without fear of making the wrong decision,
no matter how vocal and determined are the opposing forces.
The fear of the unknown tends to be worse
than the actual treatment.
Treatment for cancer has greatly improved and
survival rates are at an all-time high.
Think of the future.

How to Use This Book

This book is for women with breast cancer, their families, and others who care about them. The information in this book is based on the journalistic research of the author and is meant to educate by providing the highest quality information. To ensure that, each section has been reviewed by an appropriate health care professional. *This book should not be a substitute for professional medical care or advice.* Appropriate medical professionals should be consulted before adopting any medical procedures or treatments discussed in this book. Please understand that the author cannot be responsible for any adverse effect resulting from the use of the information in this book. Although the author has made every effort to ensure that the information presented is accurate and up-to-date at the time of publication, there is no guarantee that this information will remain current over time. Research about breast cancer is continuous and subject to interpretation.

Change can be good, and I'm not afraid to ask for help. In order to create the best possible resource for women with breast cancer, I'm interested in your comments on this book. I want to give people the best possible and most needed information about breast cancer and integrate changes into future editions and online resources.

Please send your constructive feedback and comments to:

Charyn Pfeuffer
PO Box 210601
San Francisco, CA 94121
onehundredquestions@yahoo.com

THE INTERNET

The Internet is one of the broadest sources of medical information in the world, and can be very useful when researching breast cancer. Unfortunately, it can also be one of the most confusing, overwhelming, out-of-date, incomplete, and unreliable sources. For every reputable website that contains factual information, there are others that dish out poorly referenced, obsolete, or inaccurate information. Government (websites ending with ".gov") and university-based (ending in ".edu") sites are less likely to have marketing agendas than commercial (".com") sites. While many non-profit organizations (".org") have excellent websites, an organization's political or social agenda may influence both the site's content and the sites to which they link. The American Medical Association (http://jama.ama-assn. org/issues/v285n20/fpdf/jpg0523.pdf) offers excellent guidelines for evaluating websites.

HOW DO I ACCESS THE INTERNET?

The Internet can be accessed through a connection at most businesses, libraries, and education establishments. From an initial homepage, you can endlessly travel in cyberspace. The address at the top of the screen (identified by an "http://" in front) tells you where you are. You can also type in an address of where you'd like to go. After you enter the desired address, press "enter," and the new website will appear.

DOING ONLINE RESEARCH

If you know exactly what you are looking for, you may want to use a search engine to retrieve information. A search engine will scan lists of websites to find relevant websites and specific information. When you go

to the webpage of a search engine, you will be presented with two different methods of searching; using links to topics or using a keyword search.
Commonly used search engines include:

www.google.com
www.yahoo.com
www.aol.com
www.mamma.com
www.dogpile.com
www.msn.com

ONLINE FORUMS, CHAT ROOMS, LISTSERVS, AND BULLETIN BOARDS

Forums, bulletin boards, and chat rooms are great places to share ideas
and get support, but they shouldn't be used as a replacement for medical
advice or treatment. Internet discussion groups sometimes become a place
where anecdotes and testimonials take the place of scientific evidence. Remember, every patient is different. If you hear something about a promising treatment in a forum or chatroom, take the time to research it further
in sources you know are reliable.

PART I

100
QUESTIONS
&
ANSWERS

1.

BREAST CANCER BASICS

. . . .

I find the great thing in this world is not so much where we stand, but in what direction we are moving.

—Oliver Wendell Holmes

QUESTION 1: What is breast cancer?

The body is made up of many, many types of cells. Usually, cells divide and reproduce more cells when the body needs them to repair injuries and replace worn-out tissue. This systematic process helps keep the body healthy. Sometimes, cells keep dividing when new cells are not needed, and these extra cells form a mass of tissue or cluster of abnormal cells, called a growth or tumor. Tumors can be *benign* or *malignant*.

Benign tumors are not cancerous. They can usually be removed, and in most cases they do not return. Cells from benign tumors do not spread to other parts of the body. Most important, benign breast tumors are not life threatening.

Malignant tumors are cancerous and their cells are abnormal. The cells divide without control or order, and they can separate from a malignant tumor and enter the bloodstream or the lymphatic system, damaging nearby tissues and organs. When cancer occurs in breast tissue and spreads outside the breast, cancer cells are often found in the axillary (underarm) lymph nodes. If the cancer has reached these nodes, it means that cancer cells may have spread to other parts of the body—other lymph nodes and other organs, such as the bones, liver, or lungs. The spread of cancer is called *metastasis*.

TYPES OF BREAST CANCER

Adenocarcinoma: Round or oval-shaped cancer, often clings to other tissues.

Ductal carcinoma in situ (DCIS): Sometimes described as precancerous, preinvasive, or intraductal cancer. It is noninvasive, which means it has not spread beyond the milk ducts to other parts of the breast, to the axillary (underarm) lymph nodes, or to other parts of the body. There are three grades of DCIS—low, intermediate, and high. The grade refers to how abnormal the cells look under the microscope and gives an idea of how quickly the cells may develop into an invasive cancer. DCIS is highly curable.

Medullary carcinoma: This is a type of invasive ductal carcinoma, which appears restrained but has often penetrated the lymph nodes. This cancer may grow large but has a better-than-average prognosis.

Mucinous carcinoma: This is a type of invasive ductal carcinoma, which produces a gelatinous tumor. These cancers have a very good prognosis.

Tubular carcinoma: A type of cancer that produces many small glands and tubules that closely resemble normal mammary ductules. The prognosis for this is usually positive.

Invasive ductal carcinoma: Invasive ductal carcinoma (or infiltrating ductal carcinoma) is the most common kind of invasive breast cancer and the most common type of breast cancer overall. More than half of all breast cancer cases are of this type. In more advanced stages, breast cancer cells cross the lining of the milk duct (or lobule) and begin to invade the adjacent tissues. In this stage, the cancer is called *infiltrating cancer.*

Invasive lobular carcinoma: Arises at the ends of the ducts or in the lobules and may cause widespread breast thickening rather than a distinct lump. The prognosis is better than average.

Inflammatory carcinoma: This is the most aggressive form of breast cancer. It is also the most commonly misdiagnosed, usually as mastitis or dermatitis, since the skin over the breast becomes very inflamed and swollen because the skin lymph vessels are blocked by cancer. Mammograms do not easily reveal inflammatory carcinoma, since it starts in the breast skin.

DISEASES OF THE BREAST

. . . . . .

Paget's disease: This is a very rare type of breast cancer. It appears as an itchy rash around the nipple and areola. It should not be mistaken for a skin condition such as eczema.

Fibrocystic breasts: Fibrocystic breasts are breasts that are lumpy, but the lumps are not cancerous. At the time of your menstrual cycle, one or more of these benign lumps or the general feeling of lumpiness may increase because of extra fluid collecting in the breast tissue. These lumps normally go away by the end of your period.

Fibroadenoma: A fibroadenoma is a benign (noncancerous) breast lump that is made up of fibrous and glandular tissue. It is the most common solid lump found in young women. These cysts are common and cause tender breasts, especially before a woman's period.

Breast abcess: An infection, almost always limited to nursing mothers.

QUESTION 2. What are the known risk factors?

A risk factor is anything that increases a person's chance of getting a disease. Having one or more risk factors does not necessarily mean that a woman will get breast cancer. Some women with a laundry list of breast cancer risk factors never develop the disease, while most women with breast cancer have no apparent risk factors. *Excluding gender as a risk factor, 70 percent of people diagnosed have no known risk factors.*

Known risk factors are:
- Gender.
- Earlier onset of menstruation (< 12 years).
- Later onset of menopause (> 55 years).
- Late first full-term pregnancy (after age 30).
- No children.
- No breast-feeding.
- Hereditary and family history.

- Postmenopausal obesity.
- Alcohol consumption.
- Exposure to radiation, primarily as a youth.

Suspected causes, not yet scientifically confirmed, are:
- Oral contraceptives used during the 1950s–1970s, when dosages were high.
- Environment.
- Hormone replacement therapy (HRT).
- Diet.
- Exposure to pesticides.

QUESTION 3. Who is at the greatest risk for breast cancer?

Every woman is at risk for developing breast cancer, whether or not there is a history of the disease in her family.

- Females—the single most important risk group.
- Older individuals (far more common in women 60 years and older).
- A person who has a personal history of breast cancer or who has a mother, sister, or daughter who has had breast cancer.
- Persons with a specific genetic mutation, known as BRCA1 or BRCA2.
- Women who started menstruation early or menopause late.
- Women who have never had children or have their first baby after age 30.
- Individuals who have had other types of breast disease.
- Women who have long-term use of estrogen replacement therapy.
- Women who are diagnosed with lobular carcinoma in situ (LCIS), a noninvasive growth limited to the milk lobules of the breast. LCIS is an indicator (or marker) that a woman has very high risk. Women with LCIS have about a 1 percent risk of developing invasive breast cancer in either breast per year. At 20 years, this risk is about 18 percent. There are many factors that determine the prognosis, and it is best to discuss these with your doctor.

YOUNG WOMEN AND BREAST CANCER

· · · · ·

Facts About Young Women and Breast Cancer

- Breast cancer is the leading cause of cancer death in women aged 25 to 40.
- Young women diagnosed with breast cancer face higher mortality rates, fertility problems, and the possibility of early menopause.
- Because young women typically have dense breast tissue, a mammogram is not always the best diagnostic tool for them. For this reason, and because dense breasts also make it more difficult to feel a lump, it is crucial that women ages 20 and older become familiar with their breasts and learn how to do a breast self-exam.
- There are nearly 250,000 women in the United States under the age of 40 currently living with breast cancer.
- According to the American Cancer Society, one in every 258 women between the ages of 30 and 40 will be diagnosed with breast cancer in the next 10 years.

Resources for Young Women

The Victoria's Secret Catalog Never Stops Coming: And Other Lessons I Learned from Breast Cancer, by Jennie Nash (Scribner, 2001).

Young Survival Coalition
www.youngsurvival.org
PO Box 528, 52A Carmine Street
New York, NY 10014
(212) 916-7667

The Young Survival Coalition (YSC) is the only international, nonprofit network of breast cancer survivors and supporters dedicated to the concerns and issues that are unique to young women and breast cancer.

F.A.B. (Fighting Against Breast Cancer)
www.wearefab.com
According to cofounders Jessica Mattera and Lisa Shipes, "[T]his website was designed to reach, teach, inform, communicate with, laugh, cry and share all of the experiences as women living with breast cancer. We are a minority. We are often overlooked in statistics. We are sometimes neglected in research. But, we do exist. We may not comprise the majority of new cases, but if one woman who doesn't fit the common age to get breast cancer gets it, it is one woman too many!"

MALE BREAST CANCER

· · · · ·

One percent of all breast cancers diagnosed this year will be in men. Statistically, most men are diagnosed between the ages of 60 and 70, although men can develop this disease at any age.

Male breast cancer often first appears as a small, hard, painless lump in the nipple area. Warning signs include: changes in the appearance of the skin around the nipple or the nipple itself and discharge or bleeding from the nipple. Although breast cancer is extremely rare in men, any of these symptoms justifies a visit to a doctor.

Risk Factors in Men

- Growing older.
- Family history of breast cancer.
- Klinefelter's syndrome: males with this syndrome have an extra sex chromosome and do not produce enough testosterone.
- Gynecomasta: an enlargement of the male breast; may be related to Klinefelter's syndrome, chronic diseases such as heart disease, or a variety of drugs used to treat chronic diseases.
- Testicular disorders.

Is the survival rate better for men than women?

The survival rate of men and women is comparable by stage of disease at the time of diagnosis. Men are typically diagnosed at a later stage (after the cancer has spread), because they are less likely to report any symptoms, resulting in a higher mortality rate in men than women.

Is treatment different for men?

The treatment of breast cancer in men is the same as treatment for women. Treatment usually includes a combination of surgery, radiation, chemotherapy, and/or hormone therapy.

QUESTION 4. I have heard that doctors can detect a gene that causes breast cancer. How might genes affect breast cancer risk?

While only 5 to 10 percent of all cancers have an inherited, genetic component, there are DNA tests available to diagnose gene mutations that put women at a significantly increased risk for breast cancer. The genes, known as BRCA1 and BRCA2, hold the key to genetic testing for breast cancer. Mutations of these genes account for about 80 percent of inherited breast cancers and also signal an increased risk of ovarian cancer. In Ashkenazi Jews (those of Eastern European descent) an estimated 1 in 44 carries a BRCA mutation. However, not every woman who has an altered BRCA1 or BRCA2 gene will get breast or ovarian cancer, because genes are not the only factor that affect cancer risk. Therefore, an altered gene is not sufficient to cause cancer.

HOW GENETIC TESTING IS PERFORMED

Genetic testing for cancer risk is a complex lab procedure, usually performed by analyzing a small blood sample. The test is used to determine the presence of altered genes such as BRCA1 and BRCA2, which predispose persons to developing cancer. Having a predisposition to developing cancer means that a person is at a higher risk for cancer, often at an earlier age than would be expected. Knowing if you fall into this high-risk classification for cancer may enable you and your doctor to make health care decisions to prevent or reduce your chances for cancer. Genetic testing results may be positive, negative, or uninformative and can have a significant effect on individuals and their families. Careful thought and consideration must precede the decision to be tested, and testing begins only after an informed consent process that includes a thorough discussion of the risks and benefits.

Individuals likely to benefit from genetic testing for cancer risk are those who have a family history of cancer, especially:

New information about cancer risks and genetic testing for hereditary susceptibility to cancer is announced on a regular basis. Some recent studies have found that:

- About 5 percent to 10 percent of all ovarian, breast, and endometrial (uterine) cancers are due to strong hereditary factors.
- In some families, individuals have an increased hereditary risk of several cancers, such as breast, ovarian, colon, and uterine.
- An increased hereditary susceptibility to breast, ovarian, and endometrial cancer can be passed through the father's side of the family.
- Learning about the genetic origin and risks of cancer usually reduces a person's concern about cancer.

- Relatives with cancer in several generations.
- Three or more relatives with any type of cancer.
- Relatives diagnosed with cancer before age 50.
- A relative with more than one cancer.
- Women with multiple first-degree relatives with breast cancer.

LIMITATIONS OF GENETIC TESTING

Cancer risk genetic counseling is a process of consultation with a team of health care professionals (usually a physician, nurse, and geneticist or genetic counselor). Genetic counseling before genetic testing helps individuals to make a truly informed decision about whether testing is right for them. It is important for candidates for genetic testing to consider the limitations of the test, how to cope with cancer risk, and the advantages and disadvantages of the test. Genetic counseling is necessary after testing to explain the meaning and implications of the test result.

Because testing techniques vary, it is important to know what method of testing is being used to look for a mutation and the chances of that method finding a mutation. Even with the best technology, in some cases testing may not be able to find an existing cancer-causing mutation for you or your family. If a gene alteration in BRCA1 or BRCA2 is found, there is no way to predict if and when cancer may occur.

WHAT TO DO IF YOU HAVE AN
ALTERED GENE

If you are at increased risk for breast cancer, you can make choices that may help reduce your risk of getting cancer or help find cancer early. Of course, these steps can be taken without getting tested for a BRCA1 or BRCA2 mutation.

Increased surveillance: You may opt to be monitored more closely for any sign of cancer. This may include more frequent mammograms, breast exams by your doctor, breast self-exams, and an ultrasound exam of the ovaries.

Prophylactic surgery: You may choose to have your healthy breasts removed. This surgery may reduce the risk of breast cancer.

Join a research study: You may choose to join a research study that is targeted at ways to reduce cancer risk. This may entail changing your diet, reducing the amount of alcohol you drink, or trying new drugs to reduce the risk of cancer.

QUESTION 5. Does hormone replacement therapy increase the risk of breast cancer?

Hormone replacement therapy is prescription-only estrogen or combination estrogen/progestin medication. About 20 million women in the United States are on hormone replacement therapy. It is generally prescribed to relieve menopausal symptoms (such as hot flashes, sleep disturbance, vaginal dryness, mood swings, and urinary symptoms) and to reduce the risk of osteoporosis, cardiovascular disease, Alzheimer's disease, and colon cancer. *However, research has shown that long-term use of hormone replacement therapy raises the risk of breast cancer.*

For those women who cannot or do not wish to use estrogen, other therapies are available to manage menopausal symptoms as well as disease risk. Nonhormonal therapies are available to reduce the symptoms of menopause, ranging from the use of soy products, lubricants, and vitamin supplements to prescription medications that stabilize the autonomic nervous system. Talk with your doctor about breast cancer risk before taking any hormone replacement therapy.

QUESTION 6. What can I do to reduce the risk of breast cancer?

Breast cancer is the most common form of cancer in women and the second leading cause of cancer death of women (after lung cancer). The American Cancer Society (ACS) estimated that 203,500 women were diagnosed with invasive breast cancer in the United States in 2002. An additional 50,000 women were diagnosed with noninvasive breast cancer (DCIS). The earlier breast cancer is detected, the better the chances for successful treatment. But in a perfect world we could prevent cancer from growing in the first place.

STEPS TO REDUCE THE RISK OF BREAST CANCER

- Eliminate the use of pesticides in both home and garden.
- Eat more organic food, if possible, and maintain a healthy diet.
- Replace toxic cleaners and other products in your home with healthier alternatives; a great book on reducing household toxins is: *The Safe Shopper's Bible: A Consumer's Guide to Nontoxic Household Products, Cosmetics and Food,* by David Steinman and Dr. Samuel Epstein (Macmillan, 1995).
- Stop smoking tobacco, and limit exposure to secondhand smoke.
- Stop chewing tobacco.
- Exercise.
- Limit alcohol consumption.
- Reduce exposure to UV radiation in sunlight and tanning lamps.
- Reduce fat in diet.

- Increase fiber and vegetables (although this is under debate).
- Maintain a balanced diet, including vitamins and minerals.
- Test your basement at home for radioactive radon.
- Avoid promiscuous sexual relations to reduce risk of viral sexually transmitted diseases. Human papillomavirus (HPV), a sexually transmitted infection, has been linked to cancer.

QUESTION 7. What are the symptoms of breast cancer?

Early breast cancer is usually not painful, and when it first develops, there may be no symptoms at all. As the cancer grows, the following changes may be noted: a lump, thickening, swelling, dimpling, tenderness of the nipple, or nipple discharge.

QUESTION 8. How is breast cancer staged?

Each cancer is unique, each woman is different, and the combination of treatment options is endless. To help determine the most appropriate treatment plans, doctors rely on staging, a system that helps categorize the cancer. The stage of the tumor is the most important factor in deciding what type of treatment is best for a particular case. Staging is based on three factors, known as the tumor, node, metastases (TNM) staging system:

- *The size of the tumor:* This is determined when the tumor is removed and sent to the pathologist.
- *Presence of cancer cells in the lymph nodes:* Lymph nodes are checked for evidence of tumor spread at the time of surgery in a procedure called axillary lymph node dissection.
- *Metastasis, or spread, to other organs* is assessed with bone scans, X rays, CAT scans, and blood tests (see chapter 2).

STAGES OF BREAST CANCER

There are several staging classification systems in use today. At one end of the scale are the low-risk situations: very tiny tumors that have not spread to lymph nodes. Further along are slightly larger tumors, still smaller than about a half inch (1 centimeter) and still without evidence of lymph node spread. At the severe end of the scale are the situations that involve the greatest risk: larger tumors that have invaded the lymph nodes. Tumor size is usually reported in metric measurement: 1 centimeter = approximately ½ inch. This is the scale that is most commonly used:

Stage 0—In Situ

Ductal or lobular carcinoma in situ (DCIS or LCIS), or Paget's disease of the nipple.

Stage I

Tumor is 2 centimeters (¾ inch) or smaller. Axillary lymph nodes test negative for cancer, and there is no evidence of distant metastasis.

Stage II

Tumor is larger than 2 and up to 5 centimeters (¾ to 2 inches) in size. Axillary lymph nodes may or may not be positive for cancer. If tumor is smaller than 2 centimeters and lymph nodes are positive for cancer, then the cancer is also considered stage II.

Stage IIIA

The doctor may find either of the following:

- The cancer is smaller than 2 inches and has spread to the lymph nodes under the arm. The cancer also is spreading further to other lymph nodes.
- The cancer is larger than 2 inches and has spread to the lymph nodes under the arm.

Stage IIIB
The doctor may find either of the following:

• The cancer has spread to tissues near the breast (skin, chest wall, including the ribs and the muscles in the chest).
• The cancer has spread to lymph nodes inside the chest wall along the breastbone.

Stage IV
If metastasis to other organs has occurred, cancer is considered stage IV regardless of the size of the tumor in the breast or number of axillary lymph nodes affected. Breast cancer most commonly spreads to the bones, liver, or lungs.

QUESTION 9 Where can I find a breast cancer support group or breast cancer survivor group?

A personal breast cancer diagnosis or having a friend or family member with breast cancer can often be an isolating and confusing situation. Support groups can provide a confidential and supportive forum where the many challenges of living with cancer can be shared with others.

Whether you're looking for an online support group or a local, live experience, whether you're a newly diagnosed woman or a 10-year survivor, there is no shortage of support available for women dealing with breast cancer. One of the greatest helps to healing is to know that there are thousands and thousands of other women overcoming the very same physical and emotional obstacles as you. Ask your local major hospital's breast center or departments of social work or psychiatry for support group referrals. Often, the cancer center where you receive treatment will offer support groups. County psychological associations also have divisions of health psychology, which have support groups. A college associated with a treatment center may also offer support groups. You can also call the American Cancer Society at (800) ACS-2345 for local groups that the ACS or other organizations may sponsor.

You can also look for a support group on *Breastcancer.org* (www.breastcancer.org), founded by Marisa Weiss, M.D., the founder of Living Beyond Breast Cancer and author of *Living Beyond Breast Cancer*. This website provides balanced, timely, and easy-to-understand information in an upbeat, encouraging, and respectful voice. This visually pleasing, comprehensive site will help you understand what breast cancer is, how it happens, and how it may be prevented. The always buzzing online discussion boards and live chats provide an especially warm sense of community. The best part is that if you have any questions, a real live person will respond to your concerns—and quickly.

The National Cancer Institute's website has a page, *How to Find Resources in Your Own Community If You Have Cancer* (http://cis.nci.nih.gov/fact/8_9.htm), that is an excellent starting point for finding local resources. The website includes information on Cancer, Counseling, Medical Treatment Decisions, Prevention and Early Detection, Home Health Care, Hospice Care, Rehabilitation, Advocacy, Financial, Housing/Lodging, and Children's Services. For additional support group suggestions, call (800) 4-CANCER.

The National Alliance of Breast Cancer Organizations (NABCO) has an online *Regional Support Group Database* ([888]-80-NABCO or http://www.nabco.org/index.php/20) offering support groups by state, as well as support for lesbians, men with breast cancer, and people living in Canada.

QUESTION 10. How can I receive financial assistance for breast cancer treatment?

The ever-increasing costs of breast cancer treatment can have a devastating impact on a person's financial well-being. Costs related to transportation to and from treatment, pain medication, child care, and home care can be overwhelming for patients and loved ones. The following sources can help ease financial stress by providing information and resources for limited financial grants:

- *Cancer Care's* AVON *Cares Program for Medically Underserved Women.* AVON*Cares* provides financial assistance and relevant education and support services to low-income, under- and uninsured women throughout the country. Financial aid is designated for those who are in need of diagnostic services and/or for treatment for cancer, transportation and an escort to and from treatment and/or diagnostic workups, and child care for women with families.

  Women helped through the AVON*Cares* program are able to receive services from Cancer Care. These services include: emotional support and practical assistance to women with cancer, family members, and caregivers (offered either in person, over the telephone, or via the Internet); educational seminars; and workshops (offered at the agency's offices, over the telephone, in schools, or as a part of community organizations). Cancer Care also offers information about cancer and treatment, referrals to resources in local communities for home care, child care, transportation to and from treatment, pain management assistance, and information about entitlements and breast prosthesis and wig clinics. *Mary Kay Ash Charitable Foundation Grants* are also available via Cancer Care. These grants are available for women with all types of cancer and provide limited financial assistance for transportation, home care, and child care services.

  To learn more about AVON*Cares,* Cancer Care, *Mary Kay Ash Charitable Foundation Grants,* and other services provided, call (800) 813-HOPE (4673).
- Your local *American Cancer Society* (ACS) office may offer reimbursement for expenses related to cancer treatment, including transportation, medicine, and medical supplies. The ACS also has "wig closets" where women can get a recycled wig from a previous cancer patient. Services vary by office. For additional information, or to locate your local ACS office, call (800) ACS-2345 or visit www.cancer.org.
- *Hill-Burton Free Care Program,* a national government agency, provides referrals for free medical care at participating medical facilities. Hill-Burton Free Care Program also helps low-income individuals pay their medical bills. For more information, call (800) 638-0742, or (800) 492-0359 in Maryland, or visit www.hrsa.dhhs.gov/osp/dfcr.

- *The Medicine Program,* a national nonprofit organization, provides free prescriptions for those who qualify. For more information, call (573) 996-7300 or visit http://themedicineprogram.com.
- *Pharmaceutical Research and Manufacturers of America* (PhRMA) has information about selected company reimbursement assistance programs for oncology-related products. Eligibility requirements and application procedures vary with each program. A physician or nurse can best access these programs on the breast cancer patient's behalf. Some companies offer free products for women who are uninsured and who have a verifiable financial need. For more information about the Pharmaceutical Breast Cancer Patient Assistant Program, visit www.phrma.org.

QUESTION 11. My friend or loved one was just diagnosed with breast cancer. What can I do?

A cancer diagnosis tends to create crisis, and now is the time to give your loved one a reprieve from vacuuming, carpooling, marketing, hosting holidays, and any other energy-zapping activities. Establish a "point person" who can delegate assignments to friends and family members. Have one person be an "errand person" for a day—drop off library books, buy milk, grab the mail, drive to an appointment, take the cat to the vet, pick the kids up from soccer practice, and so on. Have friends each make a dinner to store in the freezer. People want to help, but often they feel hopeless and/or helpless. By giving them a task, everyone will feel better, life will be a lot less overwhelming, and people will be brought closer together.

HOW TO TALK WITH SOMEONE
WHO HAS CANCER

Ask first.
Whatever the circumstance, whatever you want to do or discuss, the best principle to follow is to ask first. Assume you don't know what the person wants.

If the person doesn't want to talk, it may have nothing to do with you.
You can offer to listen, but that is all you can do. It is up to the person whether they want to talk to you or not.

Don't plan your responses while you are listening.
While the person is talking to you, don't mentally plan what you are going to say next. Focus on what the person is telling you.

Become comfortable with silence.

Take cues from the person.
Make suggestions, but leave decisions up to the person.

Refrain from offering advice.
Jumping in with unsolicited advice is a way of taking control over a situation. When people want your ideas, they will usually ask for them.

Be empathic, not sympathetic.
When we are being sympathetic, we feel responsible for others. We want to fix the person or the situation. It becomes exhausting. When we are empathic, we convey that the person is still in control. We empower them rather than take away their power. This feels more relaxed.

Don't be afraid to say the word "cancer."
You need not trivialize the issue, nor do you need to be maudlin. Just don't avoid the subject when it comes up.

Don't be judgmental; accept and support what they are feeling.

People react to illness in individual ways. There is no "right" way.

When the question is "Why?" the answer is "I don't know."

There may never be answers to the "why" questions. Yet the person's need to ask the questions, to struggle with them, and to try to make sense of them, is real. You may simply say that it is hard to make sense of it all.

Respect the person's spirituality.

Refrain from sharing your spiritual/religious values, while remaining supportive about the person's spiritual/spiritual values. If spiritual values come up, you can always mention that spiritual care is available.

Be yourself.

(Adapted from *When Life Becomes Precious: A Guide for Loved Ones and Friends of Cancer Patients,* by Elise NeeDell Babcock [Bantam Books, 1997].)

SCREENING, MAMMOGRAMS, & BIOPSIES

· ·

At its core, cancer prevention is not a political issue but a matter of public health and common sense. Our society is strengthened by policies that promote health and reduce disease. No matter how efficient we may become at delivering health care, we must also seek to reduce demand for healthcare services by keeping people from developing diseases in the first place.

—*Devra Lee David,* epidemiologost, visiting professor at Heinz School of Public Policy and Management, Carnegie Mellon University

QUESTION 12. Should I perform a breast self-examination (BSE)?

If you are a woman older than 20 years old, examining your breasts monthly for any unusual changes or lumps should be routine. Women who regularly examine their own breasts are more likely to notice any changes that occur. Not all lumps are cancerous, but all lumps should be checked by a health care provider. Women who are pregnant, are breast-feeding, or who have breast implants also need to do regular breast self-examinations. In addition to performing monthly breast self-exams, make an appointment with your health care provider:

- If you notice any abnormal symptoms or changes in breast health.
- If you are a woman 40 years or older and have not had a mammogram in the last year.

- If you are a woman 35 years or older and have a mother or sister with breast cancer or have already had cancer of the breast, uterus, ovary, or colon.
- If you are a woman 20 years or older and do not know how, or need help to learn how, to perform a breast self-examination.

WHEN TO PERFORM A BSE

Menstruating women experience hormonal changes due to the menstrual cycle that may make the breasts more lumpy or swollen. Women who are menstruating should perform breast self-exam from 4 to 7 days after menstruation (period) has started, when breasts are usually less tender or swollen.

Women who are no longer menstruating should do their BSE on the same day every month. Try to pick a day that is easy to remember, such as the first or fifteenth of every month, and make that the day each month for breast self-exam.

Women using oral contraceptives are encouraged to do their BSE each month on the day they begin a new package of pills.

HOW TO PERFORM A BSE

There are several techniques used to perform a BSE, and it only takes a few minutes once a month. The American Cancer Society recommends the following techniques:

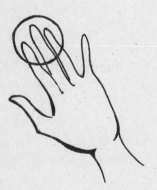

- Lie down with a pillow under your right shoulder and place your right arm behind your head.
- Use the finger pads of the three middle fingers on your left hand to feel for lumps in the right breast.
- Press firmly enough to know how your breast feels. A firm ridge in the lower curve of each breast is normal. If you're not sure how hard to press, talk with your doctor or nurse.

- Move around the breast with a spiral method, starting at the outside, working your way toward the center, or with a grid method, beginning at the top of the breast and moving linearly down. Be sure to do it the same way every time, check the entire breast area, and remember how your breast feels from month to month.

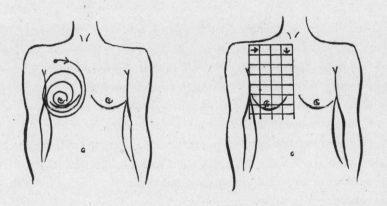

SPIRAL METHOD AND GRID METHOD

- Repeat the exam on your left breast, using the finger pads of the right hand. (Move the pillow to under your left shoulder, and place your left arm behind your head.)
- Repeat the examination of both breasts while standing, with your one arm behind your head. The upright position makes it easier to check the upper and outer part of the breasts (toward your armpit). This is where about half of breast cancers are found. You may want to do the standing part of the BSE while you are in the shower. Some breast changes can be felt more easily when your skin is wet and soapy.
- For added safety, you can check your breasts for any dimpling of the skin, changes in the nipple, redness, or swelling while standing in front of a mirror right after your BSE each month.
- If you find any changes, see your doctor right away.

BREAST SELF-EXAM
WHILE STANDING

WHAT TO LOOK FOR

- Any new lump or hard knot found in the breast or armpit.
- Any lump or thickening that does not shrink or lessen after your next period.
- Any change in the size, shape, or symmetry of your breast.
- A thickening or swelling of the breast.
- Any dimpling, puckering, or indention in the breast; nipple retraction (turning, inverting, or pointing in a new direction).
- Skin irritation or other change in the breast skin or nipple.
- Redness or scaliness of the nipple or breast skin.
- Nipple discharge (fluid coming from your nipples other than breast milk), particularly if the discharge is bloody; clear and sticky; dark; or occurs without squeezing your nipple.
- Nipple tenderness or pain.
- Any breast change that may be cause for concern.

If any of these changes are observed, women should see their physicians as soon as possible for evaluation. Rest assured, though, that in the majority of cases, breast lumps and changes are not cancer. Lumpy, bumpy breasts are by far the norm. This does not mean women should allow their fear of breast cancer to keep them from telling their physician or health care provider about a lump or change they have found.

QUESTION 13. What is a mammogram?

A mammogram is a low-dose X ray of the breast. It is used to find cancer and other abnormalities in the breast (such as cysts and fibroadenomas). A mammogram is the most sensitive diagnostic test available for early detection of breast cancer. Mammography can detect breast cancer tumors several years before they can be felt during a physical breast examination. Because it is the only relatively inexpensive technology currently available for breast cancer screening (although new technology is in the works), it is in widespread use. Mammograms are less reliable in younger women because of their denser breast tissue. And younger women, because of age alone, are at lower risk of getting cancer.

When a doctor examines mammography film, he or she will look for masses, which may be increasing in size, or areas where you may feel a new mass. The doctors are also looking for small white spots on the film, which are *calcifications*, tiny mineral deposits within the breast tissue. *Microcalcifications* are tiny (less than ⅟₅₀ inch) specks of calcium in the breast. An area of microcalcification that is seen on a mammogram does not always mean that cancer is present. They may appear singly or in clusters. The shape and arrangement of microcalcifications help the radiologist judge the likelihood of cancer being present. In some cases, the microcalcifications do not even indicate a need for a biopsy. Instead, a doctor may advise a follow-up mammogram within 3 to 6 months. In other cases, the microcalcifications are more suspicious, and a biopsy is recommended.

It is important to keep in mind that *mammograms do not prevent cancer.* Mammography is a detection device, not a prevention method. Mammograms should therefore be considered *part of,* rather than *all of,* a woman's breast health program. Mammograms should be combined with monthly breast self-exams and annual clinical exams by trained professionals.

Tip: If you've had a mammogram before, bring your old mammogram films. The radiologist can compare your old mammogram to the new one to look for changes.

HOW A MAMMOGRAM IS PERFORMED

Modern mammography has only existed since about 1970, when the first dedicated mammography imaging systems became widely available. Mammography is a relatively painless procedure that is performed by a specially trained radiology technologist. When you go for your mammogram, you may want to wear a two-piece outfit, since you will need to remove your clothing from the waist up for the exam. You may eat or drink whatever you like prior to your mammogram, but avoid using deodorant in the underarm area.

During the actual procedure, the breast is compressed between two plates attached to a specially designed X-ray machine to flatten and spread the tissue. The compression only lasts a few seconds, and the entire procedure for screening mammography takes about 20 minutes. Although this may be temporarily uncomfortable, it is necessary in order to produce the highest possible detail while also minimizing radiation exposure. For women with sensitive breasts, Tylenol can be taken 1 hour before the procedure.

This procedure produces a black-and-white image of the breast tissue on a large sheet of film that is "read," or interpreted, by a radiologist. Two views of each breast are taken for a mammogram (when no symptoms are present). Even if the results of the mammogram are not suspicious, your doctor may recommend further investigation based solely on the basis of the physical examination, as a small percentage of cancers are undetected by mammography.

Tip: When having your mammograms read by a radiologist, seek a specialist with high-volume experience. This is an extremely difficult area of radiology, and it's important to find a person with a practiced eye and some interest in the process.

SCREENING MAMMOGRAM

A screening mammogram is a low-intensity X ray of the breast that can find tumors that are too small to feel by examination. It includes two X rays of the breast—top-to-bottom and side-to-side views. It is used to look for breast disease in women who are asymptomatic, that is, they appear to have no breast problems. The results of the mammogram will show the normal features of the breast and may reveal suspicious areas that require further investigation. When you get a mammogram, you should make sure that the radiology equipment being used has been accredited by the American College of Radiology.

DIAGNOSTIC MAMMOGRAM

Occasionally, women who undergo mammography require magnification or compression views. These spot film views enable the radiologist to better view microcalcifications or small masses that are undetectable during a clinical breast examination. Often, a magnified or compression view of a suspicious area eliminates it as an area of concern, and the radiologist recommends only follow-up. A diagnostic mammogram includes two views of the breast; usually spot films that enlarge the area in question to show detail; and a sonogram to visualize the abnormality. A sonogram can help interpret if the lump is liquid (usually a cyst) or solid (benign or malignant mass).

DIGITAL MAMMOGRAPHY

From a patient's perspective, the positioning, compression, and actual machinery used for digital mammography is similar to screening or diagnostic mammography. With digital mammography, once the images have been taken they can be electronically manipulated. The physician can zoom in, magnify, and optimize different parts of breast tissue without having to take an additional image.

QUESTION 14.

What kind of risk is involved with mammography?

Mammography is *ionizing radiation*, a known carcinogen that has a cumulative effect in the body. The greater the radiation exposure or dosage over a lifetime, the greater the risk of radiation-induced cancer. This risk is highest in tissue in which cells are rapidly changing, such as the breast tissue of adolescent females. To help protect women, the Food and Drug Administra-

Carol Olby,
diagnosed age 48, DCIS

At the age of 48, I was diagnosed with ductal carcinoma in situ at almost stage II. I had complained for years of discomfort in my left breast but was told it was fibrocystic breast discomfort. Finally, when the pain went from occasional to most all of the time, I went to a woman gynecologist and she, too, felt "something." After another mammogram (which I had yearly and nothing showed up), they saw "something." She referred me to a cancer surgeon, and he declared that he believed I had cancer from only a physical exam. My husband couldn't believe that the doctor would say this after only an exam, but I knew the doctor and trusted his instincts since he had treated so many others. After having the biopsy the next day, he said he was correct.

tion (FDA) limits the amount of radiation that X rays can deliver to women's breasts to 300 millirems (a unit for measuring absorbed doses of radiation) per film, per view. In healthy women, the benefits of undergoing routine mammograms to screen for breast cancer outweigh the risks. For example, early cancer of the milk ducts inside the breast is rarely palpable but can be detected by mammography and has a very good cure rate.

QUESTION 15. What are the chances of a mammogram resulting in a false negative or false positive?

Mammography is a flawed test and misses an average of 10 percent of all tumors and as many as 25 percent of tumors in women younger than 50. Even the best and most expert mammography specialist will have a small number of false negatives. There are several reasons why a growing cancer may be missed on a mammogram. Among these are:

- Subjectivity of radiologists.
- Poor-quality mammogram.
- Interpretation errors.
- Training technologists.
- Density of breast tissue.

Another aggravation women have to contend with is a slightly larger number of false positives, in which cases they are asked to come back for a second study or a biopsy and the results turn out perfectly normal.

QUESTION 16. I do not have health insurance. Where can I get a free or low-cost mammogram?

- Medicare, Medicaid, and most private health plans cover mammogram costs, or a percentage of them.
- The State Department of Health in every state has a *Breast and Cervical Cancer Early Detection Program* funded by the U.S. Centers for Disease Control and Prevention. This program offers screening to qualified women unable to pay for it themselves. Check your phone book for listings.
- The YWCA's ENCOREplus Program has information about low-cost or free mammograms. To learn about eligibility and which YWCA facilities offer this service, call (800) 95-EPLUS or your local YWCA.
- The National Cancer Institute (NCI) can provide names of FDA-certified, accredited mammography facilities in your area. If you explain your financial situation, sometimes the facilities are willing to work out a lower fee or payment plan to make the test more affordable. Call (800) 4-CANCER for information.
- The American Cancer Society (ACS) has information about free or low-cost mammography programs nationwide and will give referrals to qualifying women. Call (800) ACS-2345 for more information.
- During October (National Breast Cancer Awareness Month), many mammography facilities offer special fees and extended hours. If you are unable to schedule a mammogram another time of year, it helps to call in September to reserve an appointment.

QUESTION 17.   What alternatives are there to mammography? Are there other diagnostic techniques?

PALPATION

The doctor can tell a lot about a lump—its size, its texture, and whether it moves easily—by palpation, carefully feeling the lump and the tissue around it. Benign lumps often feel different from cancerous ones.

BIOPSY

A biopsy is a procedure used to remove cells or tissues in order to look at them under a microscope to check for signs of disease. When an entire tumor or lesion is removed, the procedure is called an *excisional* biopsy. When only a sample of tissue is removed, the procedure is called an *incisional* biopsy or core biopsy. When a sample of tissue or fluid is removed with a needle, the procedure is called a needle biopsy or *fine needle aspiration*. (See question 18.)

ULTRASONOGRAPHY

Breast ultrasonography may be used to supplement mammography or as an independent examination. Using high-frequency sound waves directed toward the breast, ultrasonography can often show whether a lump is solid or filled with fluid.

You will be asked to remove your clothing from the waist up. Then, you lie on your back on the examining table, while a water-soluble gel is placed on the transducer (a handheld device that directs the high-frequency sound waves to the breast tissue) and on the breast. The transducer is then moved over the tissue to create an image. The test is then repeated for the other breast (if both breasts are to be scanned). You will be asked to raise your arms above your head and turn to the left or right as needed.

Ultrasonography may be used in the following types of women to detect and classify breast lesions:

- Women with dense breasts.
- Women with fibrocystic breast disease.
- Women with a lesion that cannot be well classified with mammography only.
- Young women with masses.
- Pregnant women with masses.
- Women with silicon breast implants.
- Women who refuse exposure to X rays (mammography).
- Women who should not be exposed to X rays.

NUCLEAR MEDICINE SESTAMIBI IMAGING (ALSO CALLED SCINTIMAMMOGRAPHY)

Scintimammography uses a radioactive tracer, injected into an arm vein, to identify abnormal cells on the basis of the difference in characteristics between cancer cells and noncancerous cells. The localization of the tracer can be imaged using sensitive detection devices. Normal breast tissue takes up very little tracer, which allows metabolically active cancers to be easily seen.

A nuclear medicine test is not a primary investigative tool for breast cancer but can be helpful in selected cases after diagnostic mammography has been performed. Most large nuclear medicine laboratories have facilities to perform this study, or you may want to inquire at nuclear medicine laboratories in large university hospitals.

CAD TECHNOLOGY

In April 2002, GE Medical Systems and R2 Technology were granted clearance by the FDA for the use of R2's proprietary mammography CAD technology with the GE Senographe full-field digital mammography (FFDM) system. Computer-aided detection (CAD) is used by increasing numbers of radiologists as "a second pair of eyes" when reading a woman's mammogram. This technology also is especially effective in identifying calcifications, some of which can be cancerous.

TRANSILLUMINATION AND
DIAPHANOGRAPHY

In 1929, Dr. Max Cutler was one of the first physicians to shine a light-bulb through a woman's breast. But the process, known as transillumination, produced faded images and was unsuitable for diagnosis.

Transillumination was later reborn as diaphanography. Scientists used infrared light through the breast to reveal features of the tissues inside and to try and see breast cancers, but succeeded only in detecting large tumors near the surface.

Today, scientists still use infrared light but now have the added advantage of computer programs that mathematically translate the photon pattern of the breast into an image and video cameras that are sensitive in the red and near-infrared. Diaphanography is used primarily in younger women (40 years of age or less) for whom mammography is not appropriate. It has limitations and by itself is not an adequate method of examination for suspicious lumps or thickenings in the breast.

MAGNETIC RESONANCE IMAGING (MRI)

Magnetic resonance imaging (MRI) was approved by the FDA in 1991 for use as a supplemental tool to mammography to help diagnose breast cancer. This is a noninvasive, computer-assisted technique that uses magnetization and radio frequencies to create images of the body, of the chest, abdomen, and pelvis. During the examination, the patient is asked to lie on a narrow table that slides into a large tunnel-like tube within a scanner while a radio signal is turned on and off. The energy, which is absorbed by different atoms in the body, is reflected back out of the body and continuously measured by the MRI scanner. A digital computer reconstructs these echoes into images of the breast.

This is an excellent tool for imaging augmented breasts, including both the breast implant itself and the breast tissue surrounding the implant (abnormalities or signs of breast cancer can sometimes be obscured by the implant on a mammogram). In addition to its role as a diagnostic tool, researchers are investigating whether breast MRI may be useful in screening younger women at high risk of breast cancer.

THERMOGRAPHY

Also referred to as digital infrared imaging (DII), thermography is based on the principle that chemical and blood vessel activity in both precancerous tissue and the area surrounding a developing breast cancer is almost always higher than in normal breast tissue. In this method, the temperature of the breast surface is measured. DII uses ultrasensitive infrared cameras and sophisticated computers to detect, analyze, and produce high-resolution diagnostic images of temperature variations caused by this increased activity.

There is insufficient evidence to support this method for breast cancer detection. While large breast cancers may increase the temperature of the breast, it is not proven whether small breast cancers do. Thermography is an early warning and detection system, a diagnostic tool for breast cancer, and it should be used only in addition to mammography, not as a replacement. To find a qualified thermography center nearest to you, check www.breast-thermography.com.

CAT SCAN

Computed axial tomography is the special computerized process of using computers to generate a three-dimensional image from flat (i.e, two-dimensional) X-ray pictures, one slice at a time. This method is not used routinely to evaluate the breast. If you have a large breast cancer, your doctor may order a CAT scan to assess whether the cancer is removable by mastectomy or inoperable because it has moved into the chest wall.

POSITRON EMISSION TOMOGRAPHY (PET)

This imaging is a sophisticated process that is primarily used to determine metastatic disease. The PET scanner utilizes radiation emitted from the patient to develop images. Each patient is given a minute amount of a radioactive pharmaceutical that closely resembles a natural substance used by the body. This imaging is rarely used in detecting primary breast cancer, since it is expensive and only performed in a few centers.

BONE SCAN

A bone scan is a test that finds places in your bones where there is unusually active bone repair occurring. Bone scans are most commonly done for breast cancer patients to see if the cancer has spread to bones. It is not recommended to routinely get bone scans unless there is a specific problem that you or your doctor is concerned about.

BLOOD TESTS

Blood tests help doctors detect recurrence of breast cancer in the earliest stages. Some doctors order "cancer markers" to detect possible cancer activity in the body. If cancer is present, it will usually produce a specific protein in the blood that can serve as a "marker" for the cancer. A common blood test measures CA 27-29, a tumor marker similar to CA 15-3 antigen, which found in the blood of patients with breast cancer and certain other types of cancer. As breast cancer progresses, the level of CA 27-29 antigen in the blood rises.

QUESTION 18.   What is a biopsy?

A breast biopsy is a procedure in which the doctor removes a small piece of tissue or fluid from your breast. The tissue or fluid is studied under a microscope to look for cancer cells. A breast biopsy can be done in the doctor's office, an outpatient surgery clinic, breast imaging center, mammography facility, or hospital. If the biopsy involves surgery (which occurs 10 percent of the time), you are given either a local or general anesthetic. (A local anesthetic numbs only the skin and tissues that are to be cut. A general anesthetic puts you to sleep.) Your doctor will probably do a breast biopsy if:

• You have a lump in your breast that can be felt and the doctor thinks it could be cancer.

- You have an ultrasound scan that shows a possible tumor.
- You have an abnormality on your mammogram.

Occasionally the doctor will also want to do a biopsy of the other breast or of a lymph node in your armpit to make sure that there is no cancer in these areas.

QUESTION 19. What types of biopsies are there?

The type of biopsy you have depends on the kind of lump or abnormality the doctor thinks you have. There are two basic types of breast biopsies: a *needle biopsy* (*core or stereotactic*), during which the doctor withdraws fluid or a small amount of tissue from the lump with a needle, and a *surgical biopsy,* where all or part of a lump is cut out.

Your surgeon will determine what type of biopsy is needed on the basis of whether the suspicious area is palpable (can be felt), such as a mass or thickening. Nonpalpable (cannot be felt) findings, such as microcalcifications, a very small mass, or vague density, that show up only on a mammogram also require a biopsy. More than 1 million surgical breast biopsies are performed each year in the United States. Types of biopsies include the following.

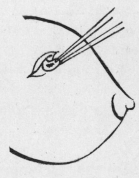

BREAST BIOPSY

SURGICAL BIOPSY

Surgical biopsies are ambulatory or day surgery procedures, performed on an outpatient basis. You will be given a local anesthetic in the area of the breast or a general anesthetic and will not feel any pain during the procedure. You should avoid taking aspirin containing medications as well as nonsteroidal (anti-inflammatory) medications for 1 week prior to the procedure. Examples of nonsteroidal.medications include Advil, Motrin, ibuprofen, and Aleve. Be sure to notify your physician prior to the procedure if you are taking Coumadin or other blood-thinning medications. You should take all other medications as usual.

Shower or bathe as usual on the day of the biopsy. Do not use any deodorant, powder, or lotion on the breast that will be biopsied. You should eat light meals and drink liquids on the day of the procedure. Fasting before the biopsy is not recommended.

A small dressing will be placed over the skin. This should remain in place for 24 hours after the procedure. To decrease discomfort, wearing a supportive bra during the day and a loose bra during the night may be helpful. You will need to limit activities that involve heavy lifting or strenuous arm movements for 48 hours. Open surgical biopsy requires stitches and a longer period of recovery than percutaneous (through the skin) breast biopsy procedures (such as fine needle aspiration, core needle biopsy, or vacuum-assisted biopsy). Usually, at least 1 full day of recovery is required.

You may develop some bruising at the site of the biopsy. Although other complications are rare, they can include infection and bleeding. The scar from a surgical biopsy is typically small. However, whether or not surgery will change the shape of a woman's breast depends on a number of factors, including:

- The size of the breast lesion.
- The location of the breast lesion.
- The amount of surrounding breast tissue that is removed in addition to the lesion.

Excisional Biopsy

Also known as a surgical or open biopsy, the purpose of the excisional biopsy is to actually remove a generous piece of tissue. The tissue that is removed is then sent to the pathologist, who performs all tests on the tissue in order to make a final diagnosis. During the procedure, the breast is cleaned and covered with special surgical drapes. Often, surgical biopsy does not require general anesthesia, and the patient will be given a local anesthetic or a combination of intravenous (through the vein) sedation with local anesthetic.

During an excisional surgical biopsy, the surgeon will attempt to completely remove the area of concern (lesion), often along with a surrounding margin of normal breast tissue. If the lesion is palpable (can be felt by examination), excisional biopsy is generally a brief, straightforward surgery performed in an operating room.

Incisional Biopsy

In an incisional biopsy, only a wedge of tissue is removed and sent to the pathologist for examination. Since most breast masses can be completely excised at biopsy, incisional biopsies are not frequently done and are usually reserved for the rare case of a very large breast mass, for which fine needle aspiration cytology (FNAC) or core needle biopsy has failed to render a diagnosis. This will then allow definitive treatment, usually a mastectomy, to be planned.

NEEDLE BIOPSY

As the name suggests, tissue samples from the breast are obtained with needles rather than through surgical methods. The advantage of needle biopsy over surgery is that it leaves little or no scarring and is less costly. The disadvantage is that compared to surgery, a needle biopsy obtains only a small portion of the abnormal tissue and can be less accurate.

The type of needle biopsy performed will depend on:

- The type of breast abnormality being assessed (the radiologist decides which needle biopsy test is most suitable).
- The skills of the individuals involved (for example, some institutions don't have a cytopathologist on staff, which eliminates the fine needle aspiration option).
- The equipment available.
- The necessity for accuracy: larger needles provide more specific information—for both cancerous and noncancerous lumps.

A needle biopsy is a simple procedure where the patient enters and leaves the hospital on the same day.

The following types of biopsies are used when a suspicious area is *palpable.*

Fine Needle Aspiration Biopsy (FNA)

This was introduced more than 50 years ago at Sloan-Kettering Memorial Hospital in New York, where it was applied to specific oncology problems. Today, FNA is an accepted method for obtaining diagnostic material from various sites, especially the breast. It is the fastest and easiest method of breast biopsy, and the results are rapidly available. This method is excellent for confirming breast cysts, and since the procedure does not require stitches, patients are usually able to resume normal activity almost immediately after the procedure.

The physician inserts a very thin needle into the suspicious area of the breast and withdraws a sample of cells from the area. This is called aspiration. A local anesthetic may be given to numb the skin. If the suspicious area is a cyst, it will produce fluid, and the cyst will collapse. If the cyst completely collapses, the fluid is discarded. If the suspicious area is solid, the aspirate usually contains cells that the pathologist can examine microscopically. Even if no malignant cells are found, a surgical biopsy may still be necessary, as cancer cells may exist in tissue not sampled by the needle. If malignant cells are found, treatment planning can begin.

Core Needle Aspiration Biopsy

This process is similar to the fine needle aspiration biopsy, but a larger needle is used, and fragments of abnormal tissue, not just cells, can be removed. When the pathologist examines these tissue samples microscopically, a definitive diagnosis can usually be made. Core needle biopsy usually allows for a more accurate assessment of a breast mass than fine needle aspiration, because the larger core needle usually removes enough tissue for the pathologist to evaluate abnormal cells in relation to the surrounding small sample of breast tissue taken in the specimen.

CORE NEEDLE
ASPIRATION BIOPSY

The following types of biopsies are used when a suspicious area is *not palpable*.

STEREOTACTIC VACUUM-ASSISTED (MAMMOTONE OR MIBB) BIOPSY

The vacuum-assisted breast biopsy is a percutaneous (through the skin) procedure that relies on stereotactic mammography or ultrasound imaging.

Stereotactic mammography involves using computers to pinpoint the exact location of a breast mass on the basis of mammograms (X rays) taken from two different angles. During this minimally invasive procedure, the patient receives local anesthesia and is positioned in an upright or facedown position. The computer coordinates will help the physician to guide the needle to the correct area in the breast.

With ultrasound, the radiologist or surgeon will watch the needle on the ultrasound monitor to help guide it to the suspicious area. Unlike core needle biopsy, which involves several separate needle insertions to acquire multiple samples, the special biopsy probe used during vacuum-assisted biopsy is inserted only once into the breast through a small 0.25-inch incision (approximately 0.6 centimeter) made in the skin of the patient's breast. The procedure usually takes less than an hour and doesn't require stitches, and the patient can return to regular activities shortly afterward.

NEEDLE LOCALIZATION

This procedure is used when the abnormality in the breast is not palpable yet the mammogram results are suspicious and require a surgical biopsy. If the surgeon recommends an excisional biopsy to remove the nonpalpable area of suspicion, then, using ultrasound or mammography, the radiologist inserts a thin needle into the breast before surgery that will guide the surgeon in locating the suspicious area for removal. Sometimes a blue dye is injected to "mark" the breast area if the margins are small. Needle localization is also called *preoperative needle localization*. An X ray is performed on the piece of breast tissue obtained during surgery to confirm that the suspicious area has been removed.

QUESTION 20.   What is ductal lavage?

Ductal lavage is a minimally invasive method of collecting samples of milk ductal cells. These cells are analyzed under a microscope by a cytopathologist who determines whether they are normal, atypical, or malignant. Ductal lavage is not a replacement for standard breast cancer detection tools such as mammography or physical exam. It should only be used as an adjunct to these methods. *It remains part of clinical research and is not a standard practice.* You should consider discussing the procedure with your physician if you:

- Have a prior history of breast cancer.
- Tested positive as a carrier for the BRCA1/BRCA2 gene mutation.
- Have determined in conjunction with your doctor that you are at high risk for developing breast cancer.

Ductal lavage involves three basic steps and can be performed in either a doctor's office or an outpatient clinic.

- *Step 1:* An anesthetic cream is applied first to numb the nipple area. Gentle suction is used to help draw tiny amounts of fluid from the milk ducts up to the nipple surface. The fluid droplets that appear help locate the milk ducts' natural openings on the surface of the nipple.
- *Step 2:* A tiny catheter (microcatheter) is inserted into a milk duct opening on the nipple. A small amount of anesthetic is flushed into the duct. Saline is then slowly delivered through the catheter to gently "rinse" the duct and collect cells. The ductal cell fluid is withdrawn through the catheter and put into a collection vial.
- *Step 3:* The sample is sent to a laboratory for analysis to determine whether the cells are normal or abnormal.

QUESTION 21. What are CEA, CA 27–29, and CA 15–3 tests? How accurate are they?

The abbreviations CEA and CA 15–3 refer to tumor markers—substances that can be detected in higher than normal amounts in the blood, urine, or body tissues of some patients with certain types of cancer. A tumor marker may be produced by a tumor or by the body itself in response to the presence of a cancer. A protein normally found in very small amounts in the blood of healthy people, CEA (carcinoembryonic antigen) may become elevated in people who have cancer or other noncancerous conditions.

Similar to the CA 15–3 antigen, CA 27–29 is found in the blood of most breast cancer patients. CA 27-29 levels may be used in conjunction with other procedures (such as mammograms and measurements of other tumor marker levels) to check for recurrence in women previously treated for stage II and stage III breast cancer. CA 27-29 levels can also be elevated by cancers of the colon, stomach, kidney, lung, ovary, pancreas, uterus, and liver. First-trimester pregnancy, endometriosis, ovarian cysts, benign breast disease, kidney disease, and liver disease are noncancerous conditions that can also elevate CA 27-29 levels.

Elevated carbohydrate antigen (CA 15-3) levels may be found in women who have breast cancer as well as in patients who have other cancers or noncancerous diseases of the breast and liver. Because CA 15-3 is seldom elevated in women who have early breast cancer, it has little use as a screening and diagnostic tool.

3.

YOUR LYMPH NODES

. . . .

QUESTION 22. What are lymph nodes?

Lymph nodes are part of the lymphatic system, which circulates a fluid known as lymph, rich in proteins and fats from the digestive tract. Lymph has its own separate circulatory system that interconnects with your bloodstream. The lymph nodes house lymphocytes that help enable increased production of antibodies. Lymph nodes enlarge during infections and if invaded by cancer cells may become infected, swollen, and tender. The lymphatic system is utilized by some kinds of cancer cells as a medium to spread through the body. The presence ("node-positive") or absence ("node-negative") of cancer in the lymph nodes is one of the most important signposts your doctor will use to determine the best treatment path with you.

Lymph nodes are oval-shaped or bean-shaped structures, contained in a fibrous capsule. Some are as small as a pinhead and others as large as a lima bean. Because lymph nodes are nested in connective tissue, they are rarely seen. However, lymph nodes are found in larger clusters in the axillary (underarm area), inguinal (pubic region), and cervical regions of the body. The number of nodes a person has varies from individual to individual.

Tumors have only three ways of spreading into the lymph nodes:

- By local invasion of adjacent tissue.
- Through the bloodstream.
- Through the lymphatic system.

Doctors are able to detect whether cancer has spread to the lymph nodes by performing a sentinel node biopsy or an axillary node dissection. With sentinel node dissection, a surgeon may have to remove only one lymph node or a small cluster of two or three nodes to know whether or not breast cancer has spread to the axilla (underarm). And this procedure leaves intact the other, noninvolved lymph nodes that perform an important function and minimizes side effects such as lymphedema, potential for numbness, heightened sensitivity, and general discomfort.

QUESTION 23.   What is node-negative breast cancer?

Node-negative breast cancer means that no cancer cells from the breast have been found in the lymph nodes (or glands) in the armpit area. If your cancer is node-negative, there is a lower risk of the cancer returning and spreading than if it is node-positive.

QUESTION 24.   What is node-positive breast cancer?

Node-positive breast cancer means that cancer cells from the tumor in the breast have been found in the lymph nodes (or glands) in the armpit area. Although the breast cancer is removed during surgery, the presence of cancer cells in the lymph nodes means that there is a higher chance of the cancer returning and spreading.

QUESTION 25. What is sentinel lymph node biopsy?

The sentinel lymph node is the first lymph node to receive lymphatic drainage from a tumor. It's named as such because the node stands "sentinel" over the tumor. The technique of sentinel lymph node biopsy spares many women from more radical surgery. During this innovative procedure, a single lymph node is removed from the axillary region (underarm) to see if it contains cancer cells. If this sentinel node does not contain tumor cells, the rest of the lymph nodes are left intact and considered free of disease. Sentinel node biopsy is gaining popularity, does not require an overnight hospital stay, and has the potential to single out affected nodes only, lessening the risk of lymphedema. Sentinel node biopsy will soon be the standard of practice.

Three methods are used to identify the sentinel node:

1. Radioactive isotope.
2. Blue dye.
3. Both of the above.

Before the actual surgery, a radioactive substance is injected into the area around the breast tumor. About an hour later, in the operating room, the surgeon injects a blue dye near the site of the cancer and uses a handheld gamma-detection probe that detects the radioactive source. The dye pinpoints only the node(s) the cancer cells drain into, and the node is then removed. The sentinel node is removed while the woman is still in the operating room and sent to a laboratory for examination. Examination of the sentinel node is performed to learn whether that node does or does not have tumor cells within it. If the lymph node turns out to be cancer free, the remaining nodes are left intact, and surgery is complete. If a woman's lymph nodes contain cancerous cells, a more aggressive treatment may be necessary.

HELPFUL HINT PRIOR TO A SENTINEL NODE BIOPSY

Many women report that the shots administered for the sentinel lymph node test are extremely painful. Ask your doctor to prescribe Emla, a topical anesthetic cream. Slather it on your breast a few hours before the procedure and wrap your breast in plastic wrap to keep the cream from wiping off on your clothing. By the time you receive lidocaine, a local numbing agent, your breasts will be numb and they will barely hurt. During the biopsy, if you still feel any pain or discomfort, tell your doctor. A considerate doctor and your insistence that you be adequately medicated will make for a more bearable experience.

Note: The blue dye will cause the patient's face to look bluish, and her urine and stools will also be blue for 24 hours.

QUESTION 26. What is axillary node dissection?

If the sentinel node contains cancer, then an axillary node dissection of the area under the arm is performed. This area is considered the initial site where the metastasis, or spread, of many breast cancers occurs. During an axillary node dissection, the surgeon systematically samples, examines, and removes several lymph nodes that normally help drain lymph fluid from the upper arm or armpit. Correct identification of these nodes can significantly improve the accuracy of selecting which to remove and evaluate for spread of cancer. It may also prevent unnecessary removal of nodes that may not be in the lymphatic drainage field of the tumor.

For many years, axillary dissection has been an important element of breast cancer management. The information gained from an axillary dissection is important for planning treatment, predicting long-term outcomes, and reducing the risk of recurrence in the armpit—all part of the disease staging process. However, a large number of women will undergo axillary dissection only to find that their lymph glands are free of disease.

QUESTION 27. What is lymphedema?

Lymphedema is a swelling of a body part, most often the extremities, but it can also occur in the face, neck, abdomen, or genitals. In mild cases, lymphedema is hardly noticeable; in severe cases, the condition results in discomfort and disability. About 7 percent of breast cancer patients experience lymphedema of the arm as a side effect after axillary dissection, making it a relatively uncommon occurrence. Radiation therapy that includes the axilla (underarm) can also result in or aggravate this condition. While most women will not experience lymphedema, the condition can develop at *any time* after surgery and, once present, rarely disappears completely.

TYPES OF LYMPHEDEMA

There are two general categories of lymphedema: primary (congenital or hereditary) and secondary (acquired). A damaged lymphatic system, whatever the cause, is unable to tolerate the demand for the drainage of lymph fluid. The true cause and predictability of the development of lymphedema remains unclear. Lymphoscintigraphy is an imaging technique used in the diagnosis of lymphedema and to evaluate lymph drainage in patients with breast tumors. It is still a good idea to be aware of the tips for prevention of lymphedema (see question 28).

Primary Lymphedema

This occurs without obvious cause and can present at different stages (see staging below). It is a malformation of the lymphatic system where lymph vessels are missing or impaired.

Secondary Lymphedema

This is a fairly common condition and may occur in people with or being treated for breast, prostate, bladder, uterine, skin, or lymphatic cancer. It may also occur after injury, scarring, trauma, or infection of the lymphatic system. According to the National Institute of Health (NIH), approximately 3 to 5 million people in the United States have this more common form. There are three stages of lymphedema. Infections are possible at any stage of lymphedema, but occurrence becomes greater as stages progress.

Stage 1 or Reversible Lymphedema (mild)
- On waking in the morning, the affected area is almost a normal size.
- There is pitting edema (when skin is pressed it indents and holds the indentation).
- There is accumulation of protein-rich edema fluid.
- Edema reduces with elevation (no fibrosis).

Stage 2 or Spontaneously Irreversible Lymphedema (moderate)
- The tissue has a spongy consistency.
- There is accumulation of protein-rich edema fluid.
- Pitting becomes progressively more difficult.
- There is connective tissue proliferation (fibrosis).

Stage 3 or Lymphostatic Elephantiasis (severe)
- Nonpitting; the tissue at this stage is hard (fibrotic) and will be unresponsive to the touch.
- The swelling is irreversible and the limb is very large and swollen.
- Accumulation of protein-rich edema fluid (a medium for bacteria and infections).
- Fibrosis and sclerosis (severe induration).
- Skin changes (papillomas, hyperkeratosis, etc.).

TREATMENT

If the lymphedema affects your arm as a result of breast cancer or its treatment, you may be referred to a breast care nurse, as some specialize in the treatment of lymphedema. In many areas, it is physiotherapists who provide lymphedema assessment

Joanne Bussiere,
diagnosed age 34, stage I

"Not enough was said to me about lymphedema before my lymph node dissection. I think I was told that there was a slight chance I'd get it. Since I didn't know what it was and no one explained it to me, I didn't blink. Well, this is a big word; it is important to understand exactly what 'chance of getting it' means. Once the nodes are removed, a woman has to adhere to a 'list' of do's and don'ts with the idea being prevention of lymphedema."

and treatment. In some areas of the country there are specialized lymphedema centers where treatment and advice are given.

If lymphedema remains untreated, it causes a progressive hardening of the affected tissues, which is the result of a proliferation of connective tissue, adipose tissue, and scarring (stage II lymphedema), and increased incidence of infection. In severe cases, a rare complication, lymphangiosarcoma, may occur. (Lymphangiosarcoma, also known as Stewart-Treves syndrome, is a rare deadly cutaneous angiosarcoma that develops in chronic, congenital nonhereditary lymphedema.)

Manual lymph drainage (MLD)

This gentle decompression manual massage technique is an effective way to activate the lymphatic system. However, if carried out as an isolated treatment for lymphedema, the results will be very temporary, and lasting evacuation of lymph fluid from a congested limb is not possible.

Pneumatic compression pump

This is a mechanical device that "milks" the lymph fluid out of the affected, swollen area. The results achieved with a pneumatic pump are usually very temporary and are of little value in stages II and III because of fibrous tissue.

Complete decongestive therapy (CDT)

This is a combination of MLD, bandaging of the affected areas, remedial exercises, and skin and nail care. Medical equipment dealers and surgical supply stores often carry products used in CDT. Elastic sleeves can be custom fitted, and arm pumps can be rented or purchased.

CDT is divided into a two-phase program that first involves an intensive treatment phase, followed by a maintenance program that the patient continues at home. Benefits of CDT: it has a high rate of success; it's noninvasive; it transfers the control back to the patient; and it is cost-effective (most insurance covers CDT).

Exercises

A lymphedema therapist will give an individualized exercise program to each patient. The exercises will improve muscular contractions and joint mobility. There will also be strengthening exercises for the limb that will reduce muscle atrophy. Muscular contractions along with the low-stretch bandages provide constant counterpressure to keep the lymph fluid moving.

Surgical procedures

Surgical procedures are sometimes suggested to a lymphedema patient. Liposuctions, superficial lymphangiectomy, fasciotomy, and microsurgical lymphaticovenous anastamoses are sometimes recommended, but no one procedure has been shown to give consistent or dependable results.

Pharmacological treatment

There are no drugs currently available in the United States to treat this disorder. At this point, there are conflicting reports on benzopyrones (Coumarin), no statistics for flavonoids (Daflon), and no evidence that diuretics will help.

Physical therapy or lymphedema therapy

Physical manipulation of the arm and lymph system by a specially trained professional may help this condition, but it is important that the professional be qualified. Many insurance plans do not cover this therapy. To find a local therapist, consult your breast surgeon, call the National Lymphedema Network at (800) 541-3259, or log on to www.lymphnet.org.

HELPFUL HINTS: *Living with Lymphedema*

Keep your affected limb warm: Make sure you always keep the affected arm wrapped up. When you are not wearing your sleeve or other compression garments, use towels to wrap and keep your arm warm.

Avoid antiperspirants: Try cornstarch, witch hazel, lavender oil, or rose water.

Tinctures: The following may be helpful: astragulus, dandelion (very diluted), honeysuckle, cleavers, horse chestnut (diluted), butcher's broom. Try adding drops of these tinctures to your bathwater and your skin will absorb the liquid. Try 5 to 10 drops a day. Remember that less is more.

QUESTION 28. How can I prevent lymphedema?

Unfortunately, prevention is not a cure. But, as a breast cancer and/or lymphedema patient, you are in control of your ongoing cancer checkups and the continued maintenance of your lymphedema.

- Avoid sunburns, burns while cooking, and harsh chemicals.
- Apply over-the-counter antibiotic on cuts to the affected hand or arm right away.
- Have all injections, vaccinations, blood samples, and blood pressure tests done in the arm not being treated/affected.
- When traveling by air, patients at risk for lymphedema must wear a compression sleeve. Additional bandages may be required on a long flight. Increase fluid intake while in the air.
- Use an electric razor with a narrow head for underarm shaving.
- Carry heavy packages or handbags on the other arm.
- Wash cuts promptly. Treat them with antibacterial medication and cover them with a sterile bandage. Check for redness and soreness.
- Never cut cuticles; use hand cream instead.
- Avoid wearing watches and jewelry on the affected arm.
- Wear protective gloves when gardening. Use a thimble if you sew.
- Use insect repellent to avoid bug bites and stings.
- Avoid tight elastic cuffs on blouses and nightgowns.
- Patients with large breasts should wear light breast prostheses (heavy prostheses may put too much pressure on the lymph nodes above the collarbone). Soft pads may have to be worn under the bra strap. Wear a well-fitted bra: not too tight and with no wire support.
- If your arm becomes red, swollen, or feels hot, contact your doctor immediately.
- Maintain your ideal weight with a well-balanced, low-sodium, high-fiber diet.

QUESTION 29. What should I ask my surgeon to see if he or she is qualified to perform a sentinel node biopsy?

- How often do you perform breast cancer surgery?
- How many sentinel lymph node biopsies have you performed, and what is your success rate with finding the correct node? (Ideally, you want someone who has performed more than 50 biopsies.)
- What percentage of the time have you been able to find the sentinel node? (You will want someone with greater than 85 percent accuracy.)

QUESTION 30. What should I ask my doctor about performing a sentinel lymph node biopsy?

- Why are lymph nodes important?
- What does sentinel node dissection involve?
- Am I a good candidate for sentinel node dissection? Why yes? Why no?
- Will you be using dye or a radioactive tracer? Where will it be injected?
- How many nodes will you remove—only the sentinel node? Or the cluster that turns blue or concentrates the most tracer?
- What are my treatment options if the lymph node shows cancer (chemotherapy, hormonal therapy, and/or radiation treatments as appropriate)?
- How urgent is it that I make decisions and begin treatment if my nodes have cancer in them?

4.

UNDERSTANDING
YOUR DIAGNOSIS

. . . .

*You gain strength, courage, and confidence by every experience in which you
really stop to look fear in the face. You must do the thing which you think
you cannot do.*

—*Eleanor Roosevelt*

COPING WITH A BREAST CANCER DIAGNOSIS

Don't ever blame yourself for developing breast cancer. Although several risk factors have been identified, no one knows *exactly* what causes this disease. Many women go through a stage of disbelief and confusion and ask themselves how this could have happened, especially if they were living a healthy life, eating the right things, and getting regular checkups. Try to limit your valuable energy going into questioning "How could this happen to me?" and remember that there are no answers and that you are not alone.

When coping with a diagnosis, there may be several emotionally challenging steps to go through, including:

- Denial.
- Questioning (Why me?).
- Fear of disfigurement.
- Fear of the treatment being worse than the disease.
- Feeling that you don't have enough information.
- Feeling alone.

It is perfectly normal for women to feel a loss of control when diagnosed with breast cancer. While the actual diagnosis is out of your control, there are many things you can control as you move through treatment. They include:

- Making educated treatment decisions.
- Restructuring your priorities.
- Learning better communication skills.
- Making healthy lifestyle changes (e.g., diet, exercise).

QUESTION 31.

What questions should I ask my doctor after a breast cancer diagnosis?

- What kind of breast cancer do I have?
- What grade is the cancer?
- How urgent is it that I make decisions and begin treatment?
- Of the symptoms I feel right now (describe them), which are likely to go away and which will remain?
- Should I stop taking hormone replacement therapy (HRT)?
- What/how should I tell my loved ones about my condition?

Kristin Young
diagnosed age 47, stage IV

"The two most important rules I live by: not only has my body undergone immense changes from the cancer and the treatment, but my mind and outlook on life have changed as well. There are many ways in which I have changed. I have become much more of a self-advocate. I have learned to appreciate every single moment of every single day. I have slowed down from 120 miles an hour to 25 miles an hour, sometimes down to 5 miles per hour. But here are the two most crucial things I have learned, and I practice them every minute of every day.

"Learn to let others help you. So many of us are supermoms or superworkers, or both. We think we can accomplish everything and take care of everyone. We are hesitant to ask for anyone's help. We wouldn't dream of asking someone to put an extra blanket on our beds. And heaven forbid, to ask a neighbor to bring some groceries over is out of the question! After a long 5 years of ups and downs, weak days and strong days, I have learned that not only is it okay to ask others for help, but it is a 'giving thing'

continued on next page

on our part to do so. Others want to help!! It gives them a good feeling to be able to help with the small things. They are happy to drive us to appointments, go to the library and bring us back a mystery, make a casserole. And we deserve it. We live in a community; we are not isolated. We like to help others. People don't like to be turned down, to be told 'No, I don't need any help' when you clearly do. We are stronger, not weaker, for realizing that. It makes us feel better, too, to realize that there are so many people in our lives who want to help in any little way they can.

"The second 'rule' that I live by is to eliminate all the negatism in my life. If that means not reading an article about how many women die each year from breast cancer, or to not take that phone call from the neighbor down the block who wants to talk about her own aches and pains, then do it. You have enough to deal with without having someone in your life who makes you feel worse. You would be surprised how many people there are who do that to us. If you stop and think about it, there's the woman from work who wants to find out how we are just so she can go back and tell others that we're really not well.

"Sometimes a negative person or thought or radio program sneaks into my life, but for the most part, I surround myself with people who really care; people who want to help; books that amuse me. I am much more able to deal with the hard things in life if I know I have only positive, loving people waiting to talk about those things when I get home. They give me hope, inspiration, and love. I feel good when I am with them."

- May I bring friends and family members to speak with you directly?
- Can you refer me to a counselor or support group specializing in breast cancer?
- Do you or your hospital or clinic have a resource center or library?
- Can you refer me to breast cancer groups or organizations in the area?
- Can you give me the name of a breast cancer expert who can give me a second opinion?
- Could you give me the names of specialists that you think I should see?
- What other tests do I need (chest X ray, bone scan, etc.)?
- What are my treatment options? How can I get more information about them?
- What are the risks if I don't get treatment?
- Can I speak with a breast cancer survivor you have treated?

COMPILING YOUR OWN
QUESTIONS AND ANSWERS

. . . . . .

Keep note cards and a pen handy (in your purse, on your nightstand, in the kitchen, in the car, in the bathroom, if you feel so inclined) to write down random questions when you think of them. Compile questions before you go to the doctor—write 'em down or type 'em up—whatever is easiest for you. Some women fax their questions in advance once they get to know their doctor. Take a friend to your appointment to transcribe answers to questions, ask for handouts, and so on. A tape recorder can also be helpful for later reference. Your elementary school teacher's mantra is true: there are no dumb questions, and it's okay to repeat the same question over and over again. Your mind is going to be on information overload, and you're not expected to remember each and every detail.

QUESTION 32. Should I get a second opinion?

Once you receive your doctor's opinion about what treatments you need, you have the right to get more advice before you make up your mind. Other doctors' opinions can help you make one of the most important decisions of your life. Getting another doctor's advice is normal medical practice, and your doctor can help you with this effort. Many health insurance companies require and will pay for other opinions.

If you have any doubts about a diagnosis or the recommended treatment, evaluate and consider all of your options. Remember that you are basically "hiring" these people to save your life, and you should be comfortable and confident with your doctors and treatment plan. Obtaining a second opinion can help you:

- Confirm or adjust your treatment plan based on the diagnosis and stage of the disease.
- Get answers to your questions and concerns, and help you become comfortable with your decisions.
- Decide about taking part in a research study of new breast cancer treatment methods (see chapter 11).

QUESTIONS TO ASK YOUR ORIGINAL DOCTOR ABOUT GETTING A SECOND OPINION

- Should I get a second opinion?
- When should I get a second opinion?
- How do I go about getting a second opinion?
- If I get a second opinion, will I have to repeat the diagnostic tests?
- Will I be able to be treated by you if I decide to follow a second opinion?

Diane Pecher,
diagnosed age 35, stage II

"There is time. You don't have to decide this instant. A couple of weeks delay will not change your condition. So you have time to ask other people. Try to find a breast center or go to a university hospital. They will have information and experts you can talk to. A good doctor will be happy to look at your case, explain things to you, and give some advice. Take your husband or another close friend with you, and think about all the things you need to ask before your appointment. You can make a list of questions. Let someone explain what the chances are that you will get cancer in your other breast. Even if your chances are increased by 100 percent, this may mean that they go from 0.1 to 0.2 percent or something like that. These are all very tough decisions, and you really need to take the time to get enough information and think about it. Don't let yourself be rushed into a decision you don't feel good about."

TO OBTAIN A SECOND OPINION

- Ask your doctor to refer you to another breast cancer specialist who is not already on your treatment team. Take along your mammogram films, biopsy slides, pathology report, and proposed treatment plan when you see this doctor.
- Call the NCI's cancer information services ([800] 4-CANCER) for help in locating cancer centers in your area.
- Contact a comprehensive cancer center near you for a second opinion.
- Talk with women in breast cancer organizations, cancer survivor groups, and other women who have been through breast cancer treatment. Keep in

mind, however, that not all breast cancer cases are the same, and individual experiences will vary from woman to woman.

QUESTIONS TO ASK YOUR DOCTOR WHEN GETTING A SECOND OPINION

- Do you agree with the original diagnosis?
- If not, what is your diagnosis and why is it different?
- What treatment would you recommend?

QUESTION 33. What is a pathology report?

A pathology report is a written description of what can be seen of organs and/or tissue removed from the body and the pathologist's interpretation of that information based on observations both with the naked eye and under a microscope. A board-certified pathologist, a doctor who specializes in the microscopic examination of tissue, should do the examination. If you had a fine needle aspiration, the pathologist may be able to identify the general type of cancer and report within an hour. If you had a core needle biopsy or surgical biopsy, it may take several days. The following information should be included in every report:

- Complete and accurate demographic information.
- Clinical information.
- Microscopic description.
- Diagnosis.
- Comments (when applicable).
- Type and relative amount of in situ disease.
- Presence or absence of lymphatic/vascular invasion.
- Tumor dimension and dimensions of components.
- Tumor grade.
- Margins.
- Presence and location (or absence) of microcalcifications.
- Nodal status and extent of lymph node involvement.

- Statement regarding estrogen and progesterone receptor (ER/PR) assay; other prognostic tests.
- Use of the pTNM pathological classification (optional).

The pathology report contains a great deal of information, but from the point of view of the person with cancer, the essential elements to clearly understand are:

- What kind of cancer was detected.
- The grade of the cancer.
- The tumor size.
- Whether the cancer is invasive and how far it has spread in the region.

The results of your pathology report will probably be ready 3 to 7 days after your surgery. This period of waiting may be one of the hardest you will face.

QUESTION 34. How do I interpret my pathology report? What does it tell me?

The first section of the report—the diagnosis section—is the most important to you, since it is a straightforward listing of the pathologist's conclusions about what he or she saw in the tissue specimens. Sometimes a biopsy is done of other surrounding organs, and a brief summary of the findings will be given here as well. The points made in the diagnosis should be well organized by number or letter, with each point specifying the name of the organ or structure removed.

At the top of the report are the basic facts about you: your name, birth date, address, doctor, and the date the specimen was received by the pathologist. It's a good idea to check that these facts are accurate. Pathology reports vary from one institution to another, but most list the final pathologic findings just below a heading such as "Diagnosis" or "Final Pathologic Diagnosis."

Following the diagnosis section is a more detailed description of the tissue specimens. This may be called something like "Summary of Sections." Here, the pathologist describes where each specimen came from and other characteristics, such as its general appearance, size, and perhaps weight. Any abnormalities found in the specimen, such as a tumor, will also be described. When a tumor is present, further tests may be done, and the results will also be included in the pathology report. If a woman has breast cancer, her breast tumor cells will probably be examined for certain prognostic indicators. The results of ER/PR assays and a HER2/neu test, if one is done, may be included as an addendum to the pathology report.

The names and titles of the pathologists who examined the tissue are listed at the bottom of the report.

> **Joanne Bussiere,**
> *diagnosed age 34, stage I*
>
> *"After my biopsy I was given a copy of my pathology report. I went over it with a friend who'd already been through this part of breast cancer. This was helpful because she explained the report to me. There is a lot of information on this report; nuclear grade (1, 2, or 3), estrogen receptor status (positive or negative), the type of breast cancer (invasive, ductal, etc.) Understanding all the terms presented gave me a greater sense of control during a time when I felt aware of my loss of control."*

QUESTION 35. What questions should I ask my doctor about my pathology report?

- What were the results of my pathology report?
- How large was the cancer?
- What kind of breast cancer is it?
- What grade is the cancer?
- Were estrogen and progesterone receptor tests done? What do the results mean for me?
- Are my liver and bone enzymes normal? ("Yes" suggests that cancer has not spread to those organs.)
- Is my complete blood count (CBC) normal? ("Yes" confirms that you don't have anemia or late-stage cancer.)
- Have my slides been reviewed by more than one pathologist?
- Can I have my biopsy reviewed by a pathologist at another diagnostic center?

QUESTION 36. What are prognostic indicators?

Prognostic indicators are characteristics of patients and their breast tumors that may help the physician predict whether the cancer will recur and plan treatment accordingly. At this time prognostic indicators commonly used are:

Lymph node involvement: Lymph nodes in the underarm and chest are a common site of cancer spread. Doctors usually remove some lymph nodes to determine whether they contain cancer cells. If cancer is found, the woman is said to be *node-positive*. If no cancer cells are found, the woman is said to be *node-negative* (see chapter 3). Women who have positive nodes are more likely to have a recurrence of breast cancer.

Tumor size: In general, patients with small tumors (less than or equal to 2 centimeters) have a smaller chance of recurrence.

HER2/neu testing: Human epidermal growth factor receptor 2 (HER2) is a gene that plays a key role in cell reproduction. About 30 percent of all breast cancer tumors are HER2/neu positive and have too many copies of this gene. In other cases, a normal number of HER2/neu genes are present, but they are a bit too bossy in instructing the cells to produce the HER2/neu protein. These cancers tend to grow and spread more aggressively than other breast cancers. They can be treated with a drug called Herceptin that prevents the HER2/neu protein from stimulating breast cancer cell growth. Knowing a woman's HER2/neu status helps a physician determine which treatments will be most effective.

Hormone receptors: Receptors are molecules within cells that recognize certain substances, such as hormones, that circulate in the blood. Normal breast cells and some breast cancer cells have receptors that recognize estrogen and progesterone. These two hormones play an important role in the development, growth, prognosis, and treatment of breast cancer. An important step in evaluating breast cancer cells is to test for the presence of these receptors. This is done on a portion of the cancer removed at the time of biopsy or initial surgical treatment. Breast cancers that contain estrogen and progesterone receptors are often referred to as ER-positive and PR-positive tumors. These cancers tend to grow less aggressively and have a better prognosis than cancers without these receptors, and they are much more likely to respond to hormonal therapy. Research has shown that about two-thirds of all breast cancers contain significant levels of estrogen receptors.

Histologic grade: This term refers to how much the tumor cells resemble normal cells when viewed under the microscope. The grading scale ranges from 1 to 3. Grade 3 tumors contain very abnormal and rapidly growing cancer cells. The higher the grade, the greater the chance of recurrence.

Proliferative capacity of a tumor (nuclear grade): This characteristic refers to the rate at which cancer cells in the tumor divide to form more cells. Cancer cells that have a high proliferative capacity are more aggressive.

Oncogene expression: An oncogene is a gene that causes or promotes cancerous changes within the cell. Research has shown that patients whose tumors contain certain oncogenes may be more likely to have a recurrence:

Ploidy and cell proliferation rate: "Ploidy" is a term used to describe the number of sets of chromosomes in a cell. Tests performed on biopsy samples are reported as: diploid, or having one complete set of normally paired chromosomes (which is a normal amount of DNA); aneuploid, or having an abnormal number of sets of chromosomes; or tetraploid, which means having two paired sets of chromosomes, which is twice as many as normal. Diploid cancer cells tend to grow slowly and respond well to hormone therapy. In general, aneuploid tumors have an unfavorable prognosis compared to diploid tumors and tend not to respond well to hormone therapy.

Other tests for predicting breast cancer prognosis: Many new prognostic factors, such as changes of the p53 tumor suppressor gene, the epidermal growth factor (EGF) receptor, and microvessel density (number of small blood vessels that supply oxygen and nutrition to the cancer), are currently being studied.

QUESTION 37. How do I tell my children about my diagnosis?

My mother broke the news of her cancer diagnosis to me over the telephone from the hospital. I had barely walked in the door after school when she called to tell me she had three months to live. The second I hung up the phone, reality smacked me in my 17-year-old face, and I began to cry uncontrollably. I knew that she was frightened (and taking a ton of medication), but to this day, I wish she'd planned her communication tactics more carefully.

There are a couple of basic tips that can help parents discuss their cancer diagnosis with their children and help ease common reactions of fear and insecurity, anger, sadness, and isolation. The dialogue that you have with your children will depend on their ages. Children of all ages can sense when something is wrong, and they tend to conjure up the worst possible problems they can imagine. Telling your child what is really going on can help ease some anxiety and fear that he or she may be feeling.

- Be sure your children have sufficient opportunities to discuss your cancer and express their feelings. You may or may not be the person they feel most comfortable talking to. They may prefer expressing their thoughts and feelings to a close friend, your spouse, a teacher, or a relative.
- Be honest with your children and provide them with the amount of information that they seek, but keep it at their level of education and understanding.
- Don't be afraid to display your emotions in their presence. This will show them that it is okay for everyone to have and show emotions.
- Provide more family time and do things together. Discuss your cancer and your feelings as a family.
- If your children respond with anger, try not to retaliate or withdraw from them.
- Be sure that children of all ages understand that they did not cause your cancer, that cancer is not contagious, and that cancer can be treated.

Carol Olby,
diagnosed age 48, DCIS

"As for telling family and friends—I just did it. My maternal grandmother died at age 52 from breast cancer, and I somehow had this gut feeling all of my life that I would probably also be diagnosed with it. Sure enough, I was, and when people asked if it floored me, I said no. I was always expecting it. But I had always thought I would never be able to deal with it. But you know? You do. It's not the end of the world; just a little speed bump in life."

- Try to change their daily routine as little as possible. Encourage them to participate in their usual activities. If possible, don't put extra work demands on them at home.
- Have your spouse or another significant person spend more time with your children.
- Once your daughter is past puberty or in high school, be sure she learns self-breast examination.

5.
TREATMENT

. . . .

We are told that, indeed, we do have cancer. Immediately, or so it seems, this calls for decisions. Do we have a mastectomy or lumpectomy, will we undergo chemotherapy and so forth. It may seem as if we must hurry up and make these choices, but hey, we just found out we have cancer. I wish I'd have thought about what I would do before ever facing the potential of cancer. Since this was not my reality, I will forever be grateful to one woman's message to me; be still and listen to your gut. I am a firm believer that in the calm the gut will guide.

—*Joanne Bussiere*, diagnosed age 34, stage I

QUESTION 38. Who should make up my treatment team?

A diagnosis of cancer may be the most difficult challenge you and your loved ones will ever face. That is why it is important to find help wherever you can and to try to maintain your sense of hope no matter what your situation. Your team of health care professionals should be knowledgeable about the many different aspects of cancer—medical, physical, emotional, or spiritual. They should be available to you as much or as little as you need. But remember that it may be difficult for them to know if you need help unless you ask for it. Don't be afraid, embarrassed, or hesitant to ask questions, voice your opinion, and seek the care you need and deserve.

Some of the medical experts who may be part of your team are as follows.

Anesthesiologist: Administers drugs or gasses, which put you to sleep prior to surgery.

Gynecologist: A physician who specializes in women's health.

Hospice care: Hospice care focuses on the special needs of people who have terminal cancer. Sometimes called palliative, this type of care centers around providing comfort, controlling physical symptoms like pain, and giving emotional or spiritual support. Hospice care is usually provided at home, although there are hospice centers that operate much like hospitals and provide full-time care.

Mammographer/radiologist: Provide mammography services for patients according to guidelines established by the American College of Radiology.

Nutritionist or dietician: Cancer and cancer treatments may cause weight loss or weight gain. For this reason, dietary or nutritional counseling or services are commonly prescribed for people with cancer. A dietitian helps to choose foods that provide the right balance of calories, vitamins, and protein to help you feel better and control your weight. He or she also gives you tips about increasing your appetite if you experience nausea, heartburn, or fatigue from your illness or treatment.

Oncologist, medical oncologist, or cancer specialist: A doctor who administers anticancer drugs or chemotherapy.

Oncology nurse: Nurses are a crucial part of your health care team, as they have a wide range of skills and are usually in charge of implementing the plan of care your doctor has set up for you. They are trained to administer medication and monitor side effects, and all major hospital centers have nurses who specialize in cancer. Whether you are staying in the hospital for care or receive treatment on an outpatient basis, you will benefit greatly from seeking assistance, asking questions, or getting tips and advice from your nurse or nurse-practitioner.

Pathologist: The pathologist is a specialist trained to examine tissues and cells. The pathologist follows a series of steps for a complete tissue analysis and uses them to make the final diagnosis. Be sure to ask if the pathologist specializes in breast cancers.

Physical therapist: A specialist who helps with postsurgical rehabilitation using exercise, heat, or massage. Ask if he or she is certified in lymphedema prevention and management.

Plastic surgeon or reconstructive surgeon: If the breast is removed (mastectomy) as part of treatment, a plastic surgeon may perform breast reconstruction. Plastic surgeons are medical doctors who specialize in surgery to alter the appearance of certain areas of the body. Plastic surgeons are certified by the American Society of Plastic Surgeons. Ask if he or she specializes in breast reconstruction.

Primary care doctor: A primary care provider is a general medical practitioner who will see adults of all ages (or a pediatrician who will see children through adolescence) for uncomplicated and common medical problems. This provider (who can be a doctor, physician's assistant, or nurse-practitioner) will often follow patients over long periods of time and refer them to medical specialists when necessary.

Psychologist: A psychologist is a mental health professional who can assist you if you are feeling depressed, anxious, or sad. While not medical doctors, psychologists have obtained a Ph.D. or master's degree in psychology and counseling; many specialize in marital or chronic illness counseling.

Psychiatrist: A psychiatrist is a medical doctor who specializes in providing psychotherapy or general psychological help. A psychiatrist specializes in helping people who are depressed, anxious, or otherwise unable to cope psychologically. Because they are medical doctors, psychiatrists prescribe medication, such as antidepressants or medication to help you sleep.

Radiation oncologist: A radiation oncologist is a medical doctor who undergoes special training in radiotherapy to become certified by the American Board of Radiology, including special instruction in the use of radiotherapy systems and other radiation therapy devices to treat cancer. Radiation oncologists are usually assisted by technologists and physicists. Ask if he or she specializes in breast cancers.

Radiation therapist: A radiation therapist is specifically trained to operate the sophisticated systems and computers used to deliver radiation therapy to the breast or other regions of the body. Typically, technologists have two or more years of training in radiation therapy and are certified by the American Society of Radiological Technologists. The radiation therapist performs the patient therapy session under the supervision of the radiation oncologist.

Social worker: Social workers are professionally trained in counseling and practical assistance. A social worker can provide you with counseling, find a support group for you, locate services in your community that help with home care or transportation, and guide you through the process of applying to the government for Social Security Disability or other forms of assistance. They also help you understand your diagnosis and talk to you about treatment side effects and what to expect. Oncology social workers specialize in cancer; most hospitals that treat cancer patients have certified oncology social workers on staff.

Spiritual support: Prayer and spiritual counseling can be very important in coping with a serious illness such as cancer. Many people find it useful to get help from clergy or other spiritual leaders, and there is no question that a strong sense of spirituality can help people face difficult challenges with courage and a sense of hope. Even if your beliefs are challenged by your illness, don't be afraid to reach out to others for help.

Surgical oncologist: Surgical oncologists perform operations to remove cancer. Surgical oncologists who specialize in breast cancer may perform breast biopsies, lumpectomies (removal of a breast lump), mastectomies (removal of the affected breast), axillary node dissections (lymph node removal), or sentinel node biopsies on breast cancer patients.

You: It may seem obvious, but it is important to remember that *you* are the most important member of your health care team. After all, it is your life and your body. As with any type of health care you receive, you are a consumer of services. You should feel empowered to ask questions about what treatment you are getting, who is providing it, and where you can find more information about what you're discussing. Although your treatment team is committed to making you disease free, it's up to you to do some homework to make the most informed and best decisions for you. It has been shown that patients who are empowered with awareness of their disease, treatment options, and tools for self-care make healthier choices in the management of their breast cancer.

QUESTION 39. How do I select the members of my treatment team?

To find a surgeon: Ask your family doctor or gynecologist for a referral. Your doctor can also contact the American Society of Clinical Oncology (ASCO) for referrals to local surgical oncologists who are ASCO members. The American Board of Medical Specialists, at (800) 776-2378, can verify a physician's board certification by specialty and year and will refer callers to local board-certified doctors.

To find a plastic surgeon: To verify that a plastic surgeon for corrective or reconstructive surgeries is certified, or to check credentials, call the American Society of Plastic and Reconstructive Surgeons referral service at (800) 635-0635.

To find a medical or radiation oncologist: Oncology is the study of tumors. *Medical oncologists* are physicians who specialize in treating cancer

Eric Winer, M.D., *director of the Breast Oncology Center at Dana-Farber Cancer Institute and associate professor of medicine at Harvard Medical School (at the 2001 San Antonio Breast Cancer Symposium)*

"When you're healthy and you don't have any medical problems, your relationship with your doctor and nurses doesn't make a lot of difference. But when you have an illness, the relationship with the health care team plays a much bigger role. When people have medical problems like breast cancer, they need to get care they're comfortable with."

with medicine/chemotherapy. *Radiation oncologists* are physicians who specialize in treating cancer with therapeutic radiation. The American Society of Clinical Oncology's website, www.asco.org, has an oncologist locator service that includes all of ASCO's 17,000 members; ASCO can also be reached at (703) 299-0150.

When selecting either a medical or radiation oncologist, it is important to find a facility that handles a large volume of patients and that conducts research (particularly clinical trials), and an oncologist who has considerable experience in the treatment of breast cancer and who is either an ASCO member or active member in another professional society in the field of clinical oncology. If you live in a town where the oncologist, who may the best and the brightest, treats only a handful of breast cancer patients a year, it may be beneficial to make the road trip to someone with more experience. Compassion is an important aspect of treatment, but it's a doctor's technical expertise that will save your life.

To find a nurse: Call Ask-A-Nurse, a free service providing 24-hour health care information and referrals from registered nurses in select locations around the country. Call (800) 535-1111 to find out if there is an office in your area.

To find a clinical or comprehensive cancer center: Call the National Cancer Institute's cancer information service at (800) 4-CANCER for the names of NCI-affiliated clinical or comprehensive cancer centers in your state or members of the NCI's Community Clinical Oncology Program (CCOP).

QUESTION 40. What are the most common treatments for breast cancer?

Breast-conserving surgery (BCS): Removes the cancerous lump in the breast and some of the surrounding tissue. The surgery is usually followed by radiation therapy. A mastectomy is the removal of the entire breast plus surrounding lymph nodes. See chapter 6.

Radiation therapy: Uses high-dose radiation to kill the cancer cells. Usually used following surgery to control any remaining tumor and to reduce the chance of recurrence. See chapter 7.

Chemotherapy: Uses drugs to kill cancer cells. See chapter 8.

Hormonal therapy: Uses drugs that change the way hormones work or removes the organs that produce hormones, such as the ovaries. Chemotherapy and hormonal therapy can be used together to lessen symptoms if the cancer has spread. See chapter 9.

QUESTION 41. What does "drug treatment" mean?

Drug treatment can mean either chemotherapy or hormonal therapy.

QUESTION 42. What is radiofrequency ablation?

This is an experimental technique that uses heat, similar to that generated by a microwave, to "burn" away tumors. The technique may be an effective method of treating small breast cancers, according to a report in the January 2002 issue of *American Surgeon*, and may allow some patients with small tumors to avoid surgery.

Normally, doctors would perform a lumpectomy to surgically remove the cancerous tissue, but radiofrequency ablation has shown promising results. More studies are needed to determine the protocol of the new technique, but researchers are optimistic because:

- Radiofrequency ablation is less risky than surgical removal or biopsies.
- No major side effects and little pain were reported during or after the procedure.
- The technique is suitable for use on tumors too small to be visualized by ultrasound methods.
- It's a cost-effective technique, because it's done without general anesthesia in an outpatient or office setting.

QUESTION 43. What factors does my doctor consider when recommending my treatment plan?

Your doctor will prescribe a treatment plan that could include any combination of surgery, radiation, chemotherapy, or hormone therapy, depending on:

- Type of tumor.
- Size of the tumor.
- Size of your breast.
- Location of the tumor in your breast.
- Possibility of spread of cancer to lymph nodes or to skin, muscle, chest wall, bone, or other organs.
- Appearance of your mammogram.
- Your desire for immediate or future reconstruction.
- Your general health.
- Which surgery will give you the best chance for survival.
- Which surgery will give you the best cosmetic results.
- Which surgery will give you the best use of your arm afterward.
- Results of studies made on the tumor (for instance, if hormones promoted its growth, how fast it is growing) and results of other tests.
- What your priorities are for surgery.

QUESTION 44. How does my doctor determine the order in which I receive treatment?

Until recently, women weren't offered much beyond "slash, burn, and poi-son," or what is more commonly referred to as surgery, radiation, and chemotherapy. While these are still the standard methods of treatment, women now have more choices.

Breast cancer is almost always treated with breast surgery. Depending on your type and stage of cancer, your doctor may recommend one kind of surgery, or you may have a choice. There are two basic kinds of surgery used to treat breast cancer: mastectomy and lumpectomy (or breast-conserving surgery).

After a lumpectomy, radiation treatment kills any cancer cells that might be left in the breast after surgery.

Chemotherapy drugs kill cancer cells that may have spread in the body. While surgery treats the breast, chemotherapy can treat the whole body. Some people need chemotherapy to treat their cancer; others do not. Chemotherapy can help reduce the chance of breast cancer coming back after surgery. It can be given before or after surgery, depending on the size and kind of breast cancer. Your doctor may give you more than one drug. Some are given in pill form; most are injected.

Doctors now use special drugs known as "hormone blockers" to pre-vent the natural hormones in your body from attaching to cancers, so the cancer cannot grow. Doctors may use these drugs to treat early and ad-vanced breast cancers. If you have had cancer in one breast, these drugs may help prevent new cancers from growing in a different spot in your breast or from growing in your other breast. These drugs are given as a pill, which is usually taken every day for several years.

QUESTION 45. What are my treatment options if I am diagnosed with breast cancer while pregnant?

A diagnosis of breast cancer is traumatic for any woman, but even more so if it overlaps with pregnancy. Luckily, the combination is relatively rare, occurring in approximately 3 out of every 10,000 pregnancies.

Detecting breast cancer in women who are pregnant, nursing, or have just given birth can be difficult. During pregnancy and while a mother is nursing, the breasts are tender and swollen, making small lumps difficult to detect. With an increased probability of delayed detection, cancers are often found at a later stage in these women.

Surgery is usually recommended as the primary treatment of breast cancer in pregnant women. First-trimester radiation therapy should be avoided, since it may expose the fetus to potentially harmful radiation. Modified radical mastectomy is the alternative treatment of choice, and postpartum radiation therapy is used for breast preservation. Chemotherapy can be given in the second or third trimester, or, for women who want to save their breast, chemotherapy can be given before surgery and radiation would be delayed until after delivery.

Overall survival of pregnant women with breast cancer may not be as good as nonpregnant women at all stages, most likely because of delayed diagnosis. No damaging effects on the fetus from maternal breast cancer have been confirmed.

QUESTION 46. What questions should I ask my doctor about starting breast cancer treatment?

- How will your age, sex, and overall health affect the outcome?
- What is the diagnosis of your disease? What are the grade and stage of the disease?
- How will any prior therapy affect current therapy attempts?
- What are the documented statistics for "success" with this form of therapy, particularly for comparable individuals (same sex, age, type and grade of tumor, stage of cancer)? And by "success" is the doctor referring to increased longevity, reduction in tumor size, no detectable tumor, or something else? And for how long?
- What are the documented percentages of people on this particular therapy who have encountered adverse side effects (hair loss, nausea, pain, loss of weight, headaches, lethargy, increased likelihood of an infection, etc.)?
- How advanced is your form of cancer? Has it metastasized?
- What will your quality of life be during and after therapy?
- Does the doctor have easy-to-understand literature available for you to read concerning this therapy, prior to commencing treatment?
- For individuals of child-bearing age, what is the potential impact on fertility or your ability to have children after therapy?
- What other types of medicines are available to help you through the cancer treatment (e.g., painkillers, antinausea drugs, etc.)?
- Where will the therapy be performed? Will it require frequent long-distance travel? Do you have a support partner or organization?
- Should you consider experimental, alternative, or complementary therapies? If so, where are the centers of excellence located for each? Is there any scientific evidence that these options might work?
- What are the financial costs? What portions of your bills will not be covered by your insurance, Medicare, your employer, and so on?
- How many options do you have (chemotherapy, surgery, alternative medicine, palliative care/assistance with pain management, prayer, etc.)?

6.

MASTECTOMY, LUMPECTOMY, & BREAST RECONSTRUCTION

. . . .

QUESTION 47. What is mastectomy?

Mastectomy is the surgical removal of the breast for the treatment or prevention of breast cancer. There are several types of mastectomy:

- **Total or simple mastectomy** is the removal of the whole breast, and no lymph nodes under the arm are removed.
- **Subcutaneous mastectomy** is when the tumor and breast tissue are removed, but the nipple and the overlying skin are left intact. Reconstruction surgery is easier, but some cancer cells may remain.
- **Modified radical mastectomy** is the removal of the breast and many of the lymph nodes under the arm.
- **Radical mastectomy** (or the **Halsted technique**) is the removal of the breast, chest muscles, and all of the lymph nodes under the arm. This procedure is rarely performed, and only in situations where the tumor has spread elsewhere.
- **Skin-sparing mastectomy** is a relatively new surgical procedure that may be an option for some patients. During this procedure, the surgeon makes a much smaller incision, sometimes called a "keyhole" incision, circling the areola. Even though the opening is smaller, the same amount of breast tissue is removed. Scarring is minimal, and 90

percent of the skin is preserved. Reconstruction is performed at the same time as the procedure by a plastic surgeon, using tissue from the patient's abdomen or latissimus dorsi, a muscle in the back.

QUESTION 48. What is a lumpectomy?

A partial or segmental mastectomy involving the removal of the breast tumor (usually a cancer), as well as a wide surrounding margin of breast tissue around the tumor, is known as a lumpectomy. The definition of "wide" is somewhat variable, but most surgeons attempt to remove at least 2 centimeters of surrounding breast tissue around the tumor and leave the remaining breast tissues, the nipple, and the areola intact. Usually, some of the lymph nodes under the arm are taken out. In most cases, radiation therapy follows. After surgery, you do not have to wear a prosthesis or special bra as you would after a mastectomy. There are some reasons why you may not be a candidate for a lumpectomy, such as being pregnant or having multiple tumors.

Advantages
As effective as mastectomy.
Breast is spared.
Preserves normal nipple and skin sensation.
Usually yields good cosmetic results.

Disadvantages
Not an option for women whose bodies are too sensitive for radiation therapy. (Such women might have certain connective tissue disorders or Hodgkin's disease or be pregnant.)

HELPFUL HINT: *What to Wear*

If you must wear a bra after your lumpectomy or lymph node dissection, many women report that Lane Bryant (www.lanebryant.com) makes a super-comfy T-shirt bra. And shirts and blouses that button in the front eliminate the difficult task of trying to maneuver a top over your head. Button-down tops also make access to drains much easier.

QUESTION 49. Do I have a choice between mastectomy and lumpectomy?

In most cases, both surgeries have been proven to have equal survival rates and are equally effective in treating breast cancer. There are advantages and disadvantages to each. You need to evaluate which procedure best suits your lifestyle. The decision can be hard, and you may want to talk to patients who have had each type of surgery if you are having problems evaluating which is best for you. Ask your surgeon for the name of a peer, or call the American Cancer Society and ask for a Reach To Recovery volunteer who will talk to you about her choice of surgery. Talk to mastectomy and lumpectomy surgical patients to help with your decision. Sometimes a woman chooses lumpectomy, but the surgeon, while operating, finds more tumor than expected. In this case, the woman will need a reexcision or possibly a mastectomy in the future. However, many women have the choice. They can, and should, choose the one that is better for them.

QUESTION 50.   What factors should I consider in choosing between mastectomy and lumpectomy?

The factors that women consider in making this decision are the same re-gardless of which option they choose. These factors include:

- Fear of recurrence.
- Avoiding a possible second surgery.
- Physician's preference or recommendation.
- Appearance and body image.
- Side effects of radiation.
- Fear of radiation.
- Inconvenience of radiotherapy.
- Experiences of other women.
- Feelings of their partner or others.
- The importance for them, of keeping their breast.
- Arm mobility.
- Breast reconstruction.
- Amount of pain.
- Effect on survival.
- Ability to have radiation treatment 5 days per week for several weeks.
- Association of breasts with sexuality.

QUESTION 51.   Do I need radiation therapy if I have a lumpectomy?

Radiation therapy is almost always given following a lumpectomy to de-stroy any abnormal cells that may remain elsewhere in the breast. Radiation therapy is one reason why lumpectomy is so successful at treating breast cancer.

QUESTION 52. Is it possible to have a lumpectomy even if I can't have radiation treatment afterward?

A lumpectomy without radiation is not currently recommended because the tendency for cancer to recur is higher. The only exception is patients with very tiny amounts of DCIS. There is currently a clinical trial for this.

QUESTION 53. If I have a lumpectomy followed by radiation treatment, can the cancer still come back?

Studies have demonstrated that patients with breast cancer have the same survival rate if they are treated with a lumpectomy and radiation as with a mastectomy.

There is little question that breast radiation reduces local recurrence after lumpectomy, and this reduction is important if one of the goals of the clinic is breast preservation. A recent study showed that in women with small tumors treated with lumpectomy alone for clear margins and followed along with regular visits to the doctor without undergoing radiation treatments, recurrence of the disease in the breast that had the cancer surgically removed was 20 percent within 66 months of follow-up.

QUESTION 54. What if the tumor is right next to or involving the nipple?

Cancers located in the central portion of the breast, behind or near the nipple, present a challenge. Lumpectomy in these cases usually requires removing the entire nipple and areola as part of the lumpectomy. In this case, an incision is made around the nipple, to incorporate the nipple and areola with the underlying breast specimen. This is necessary to ensure that a complete margin is taken around the cancer. Simply cutting under the nipple and areola would result in a loss of blood supply to those structures, and subsequent tissue death (necrosis). In this type of lumpectomy, a plastic surgeon will usually perform a reconstruction of the nipple and areola later. Because cancers behind or near the nipple require this special type of lumpectomy, the cosmetic outcome may be harder to predict. Therefore, many surgeons and radiation therapists are uncomfortable with conservative therapy of breast cancer in this location.

QUESTION 55. After a mastectomy, can I have my breast reconstructed?

Breast reconstruction is a surgical procedure for women with breast cancer that rebuilds the breast contour and, if the women wishes, the nipple and areola. There are two different types of reconstruction procedures—an *implant* and a *muscle flap*. The choice depends on the amount and suitability of tissue remaining at the surgery site, the desire to match the opposite breast, the recovery time, and the possible loss of muscle function. Breast reconstruction is most often an option for a woman who has had a mastectomy and whose entire breast has been removed. In some cases, reconstruction cannot be done because of the aggressiveness of disease.

Breast reconstruction will restore your body image after a mastectomy and prevent you from having to wear a prosthesis (breast form) and special bras. Reconstructive surgery may be performed at the time of your mastectomy, after treatment for your cancer is completed, or even years later. Both immediate and delayed reconstruction have advantages and disadvantages to consider. You should look at your options closely before you have any surgery. Even if you choose delayed reconstruction, this decision is best made before any surgery to ensure that your later option for reconstruction will not be impaired. Age is not a factor in a woman having reconstruction. However, general health is a vital consideration at any age. Women who have mastectomies and choose reconstruction are usually very pleased with the results. If

BREAST RECONSTRUCTION OPTIONS

	PROSTHESIS	IMPLANT	
Who is a candidate?	All women	Small-breasted women	
Timing	During the initial recovery period, a lightweight style is best. After the mastectomy scar heals, a more lifelike silicone model can be used.	Immediate or delayed	
Length of recovery	None	3 to 4 weeks before returning to work or performing strenuous activities	
Scarring	Mastectomy scar	Mastectomy scar	
Drains	Drains from mastectomy only	Worn for between 3 days and 2 weeks after surgery (1 week average)	
Hospital stay	Hospital stay for mastectomy only (outpatient to 2 days)	1 to 2 days if immediately following mastectomy; outpatient to 1 day if delayed	
Follow-up	None	Additional surgeries possible to remove or repair implant	
Possible complications	Adapting swimsuits and lingerie to hold the prosthesis, self-conscious feeling in clothes, sweating under prosthesis, unreachable itches	Implant may leak, harden, or become infected	

TISSUE EXPANDER	NATURAL TISSUE TRAM FLAP	NATURAL TISSUE LATISSIMUS DORSI
Most women	Most women	Most women
Immediate or delayed	Immediate or delayed	Immediate or delayed
3 to 4 weeks before returning to work or performing strenuous activities	6 to 8 weeks before resuming normal activities	4 to 6 weeks to return to work and resume normal activity
Mastectomy scar	Scarring at donor site on the abdomen (hip to hip); mastectomy scar	Scarring at donor site on the back; mastectomy scar
Worn for between 3 days and 2 weeks after surgery (1 week average)	Worn for 3 days to 3 weeks after surgery (1 week average)	Worn for 3 days to 3 weeks (1 week average)
1 to 2 days if immediately following mastectomy; outpatient to 1 day if delayed	3 to 5 days	3 to 5 days
Additional surgeries required to remove tissue expander and to insert implant. Further surgeries if complications with implant	Additional surgeries possible for additional contouring or to correct complications	Additional surgeries possible to remove or repair implant
Tissue expander may leak or become infected; implant may leak, harden, or become infected	Hernia; potential loss of abdominal wall strength; changes overall body appearance; potential loss of reconstructed breast	Potential loss of reconstructed breast; implant complications

you are considering immediate reconstruction, it is important to keep in mind: you won't have to wake up from surgery without a breast, and one surgery (vs. two) means lower medical costs, fewer possible complications from anesthesia and surgery, and a shorter overall recovery time. If you are considering waiting on reconstruction, keep in mind that you have additional time to make reconstruction decisions; for women undergoing chemotherapy, it possibly lessens the chance of infection in the reconstruction site; and that it avoids scheduling snafus in coordinating operation efforts.

QUESTION 56. How do I choose my plastic surgeon?

Breast reconstruction is not an emergency procedure. Take your time to consider your options, and shop around for the best plastic surgeon. It is important to consult with your breast surgeon for a referral. Make sure that any plastic surgeon you consider is board certified in plastic surgery and is experienced, if not a specialist in breast reconstruction. The American Society of Plastic Surgeons (ASPS) can tell you if a specific surgeon is board certified. Call (800) 635-0635.

QUESTION 57. Will breast implants interfere with mammograms?

While there is no evidence that breast implants cause breast cancer, they may change the way mammography is done to detect cancer. When you request a routine mammogram, be sure to go to a radiology center where technicians are experienced in the special techniques required to get a reliable x-ray of a breast with an implant. Additional views will be required. Ultrasound examinations may be of benefit in some women with implants to detect breast lumps or to evaluate the implants.

Silicone breast implants are also known to be associated with calcium deposits in the breast. These calcium deposits can make it even more difficult to obtain a clear mammogram than it already is. However, in general, calcium deposits can be indicative of a nearby cancer. Therefore, the presence of silicone implants may make it difficult to determine if there is cancer present or if all the mammogram is showing are the effects of the implants.

Breast self-exams are also muddled by implants. Implants, put under the chest muscle, can make it difficult to feel the breast tissue properly. In addition, calcium deposits or hardening of saline implants can cause lumps to appear in the breast that are not associated with cancer. This can confuse matters and cause undue worry.

If you get implants postmastectomy, mammograms are no longer performed.

QUESTION 58. What questions should I ask my doctor about mastectomy, lumpectomy, breast reconstruction, and implants?

- What are the board certifications of the surgeon performing the procedure?
- What should I do to prepare for my surgery?
- Is lumpectomy an option for me? Why or why not?
- How much breast tissue will be removed?
- Where and how big will the scar be?
- Will you remove any of my lymph nodes?
- If I am advised to have a mastectomy, what are the risks and benefits of immediate breast reconstruction? What are my reconstruction options?
- Does a mastectomy decrease the chance of recurrence?
- How will my breasts look after the treatment? Do you have photographs?
- Can breast reconstruction be done at the time of my mastectomy or should it be done later?
- Can you refer me to a plastic surgeon so I can discuss my reconstruction options?

- What type of reconstruction do you think is best for me?
- Will an implant make it more difficult to detect a local recurrence?
- Will a nurse or physical therapist teach me to care for and exercise my arm after surgery?
- Will my insurance cover reconstruction, even if it's done later? Will it cover breast prosthesis?
- Do you have a peer referral with whom I can discuss my concerns about the procedure and recovery?

With all procedures, it's important to ask:

- How much pain should I expect in the days following the procedure?
- Should I arrange to have someone help me with daily activities?
- What is the expected recovery period? When will I be able to resume normal activities, and which activities should I avoid?
- Will there be any long-term effects I should be aware of?

QUESTION 59. What questions should I ask my doctor about pain relief?

- How much pain should I expect in the days following the procedure?
- What can I do to relieve the pain?
- How and when should I take the medicine(s) and for how long?
- What side effects are common? What should be done if they occur?

RADIATION THERAPY

· ·

QUESTION 60. What is radiation
therapy? What are the
different kinds of
radiation therapy?

Radiation therapy is the treatment of disease using penetrating beams of
high-energy waves or streams of particles called radiation. Radiation is in
every part of our lives. It occurs naturally in the earth and can reach us
through cosmic rays from outer space. Radiation may also occur naturally
in the water we drink or the soils in our backyard. It even exists in food,
building materials, and in our own human bodies. We can also come into
contact with radiation through sources such as X rays, nuclear power plants,
and smoke detectors.

    At high doses, radiation is used to treat cancer and other illnesses. Radi-
ation therapy may be used alone or in combination with chemotherapy or
surgery. The actual radiation treatments are painless.

WHAT TO EXPECT

The radiotherapy machine is a large piece of equipment housed in its own special room, often at basement level. This is so that the radiotherapy can be given safely to you, while not exposing anyone else unnecessarily to radiation. Each treatment lasts only for a few minutes and is not painful. You will lie on a hard couch under an X-ray machine and will not feel the treatment taking place. The machine may make a slight noise.

Before the first treatment, the chest is marked with ink or a few long-lasting tattoos. These marks must stay on the skin during the weeks-long course of treatment because they indicate the precise location where the radiation beams must be placed. The radiation oncologist plans specific treatment based on a physical exam, mammograms, pathology laboratory reports, and that patient's state of health throughout the therapy. Each treatment last about 20 to 25 minutes, but the breast is only exposed to high-energy X rays for a few minutes. It's good to allow 30 minutes for each treatment to be safe. Most of the time is spent positioning the patient for the best results.

TYPES OF RADIATION

Like all aspects of modern medicine, the field of therapeutic radiology continues to make advances in knowledge and technology. Many new variations of radiation treatment are being used and studied to find more effective treatments for cancer.

External beam radiotherapy uses high-energy rays, usually X rays or photons, which are sometimes called "packets of energy," to kill cancer cells. The higher the energy of the X-ray beam, the deeper the X rays penetrate into the target tissue. It is a localized treatment, meaning it kills cells only in the area of the body that it is pointed at and nowhere else. Cancer cells are more sensitive to radiotherapy than normal cells and more will be killed. Normal cells that are affected usually recover or repair themselves quite quickly.

Gamma rays are another form of photon used in radiotherapy. Gamma rays are produced spontaneously as certain elements (such as radium, uranium, and cobalt 60), which release radiation as they decompose, or decay. Each element decays at a specific rate and gives off energy in the form of gamma rays and other particles. X rays and gamma rays have the same effect on cancer cells.

Internal radiotherapy or **brachytherapy** is a way of giving radiation treatment internally. Breast cancer doctors have been using brachytherapy as a follow-up to lumpectomy. It works from the inside, with radioactive "seeds" injected into the breast at the site of the excised tumor, where cancer is most likely to recur. The entire treatment takes about 5 days instead of 5 to 7 weeks. Because the treatment is so short, the brachytherapy can be given before chemotherapy is started (if chemotherapy is required).

Investigational techniques include the following:

Intraoperative irradiation is the use of external beam radiation therapy during surgery to treat cancerous tumors or certain other forms of cancer. Intraoperative irradiation, when used in conjunction with surgery, external beam therapy, and/or chemotherapy, has been shown to improve the outcome of cancer treatment in certain situations. Benefits of intraoperative irradiation include a decreased area of irradiated tissue, as the target area is directly visible, and a more effective dose of radiation may be used.

Three-dimensional (3D) conformal radiation therapy: Protocols and techniques for this therapy are being developed and refined to improve the application and outcomes of radiation therapy.

Particle beam radiation therapy is the use of higher-energy radiation particles in cancer therapy. This type of radiation therapy offers benefits related to the individual cells under treatment. Two types of particle radiation therapy are under study: *fast neutron therapy* and *charged particle therapy*. Fast neutron therapy may be used in the treatment of certain inoperable or recurrent tumors. Because of the cost of the equipment and the need for improved technology, there are only three centers in the United States and 10 centers in the entire world that offer fast neutron therapy. There are a few more centers offering charged particle therapy. However, only a small number of patients have been treated with this type of radiation therapy.

Thermoradiotherapy (hyperthermia) is the use of heat at the site of treatment. It has been shown experimentally to improve the response of certain cancers to other forms of radiotherapy, as well as to chemotherapy.

QUESTION 61. Why is radiation necessary after a lumpectomy?

Radiation therapy is performed after lumpectomy to help ensure that no cancer cells that may have escaped surgical removal survive in the breast.

QUESTION 62. How soon after my lumpectomy must I start radiation therapy?

Barbara McCoart,
diagnosed age 48, stage IV

"As for the radiation, it was a relaxing time for me. I would let my mind think about all the great things I would do when all my treatments were over. Cancer is not a death sentence, and you will have a wonderful life that will feel much fuller and much more meaningful once all this is over. Just learn to take each day and live it for all it's worth, and plan for a wonderful future, because we do have futures, and my future is much more spiritual and meaningful than it ever was before my cancer."

Women who have lumpectomy typically begin outpatient radiation treatment 4 weeks after surgery, with brief treatments 5 days a week for 6 weeks. Each treatment lasts about 20 to 25 minutes, but the breast is only exposed to high-energy X rays for a few minutes. Many lumpectomy patients receive a booster dose of radiation to the area where the lump was located. This time commitment can be discouraging for women with transportation difficulties or lack of time, or who live a distance from the treatment facility.

QUESTION 63. What are the side effects of radiation therapy, and how long do they last?

Common short-term side effects are fatigue and skin irritation known as *radiation erythema*. Long-term changes include change in size and color of breast or a feeling of heaviness. Luckily, side effects of radiation are usually temporary.

Skin changes that occur may vary from no changes to a dry, scaly, pink color to a bronzed reddening of the skin, varying amounts of swelling, and production of free radicals. The sebaceous glands that lubricate the skin in the treated area may decrease productivity posttreatment, causing excessively dry skin. Skin reactions may be more severe if you are receiving chemotherapy and radiation therapy at the same time but will usually subside 2 to 4 weeks after the treatment course is completed. Here are some women-recommended products that will protect and soothe the skin during and after radiation treatments:

Clinique Moisture Surge Extra Thirsty Skin Relief: www.clinique.com, or available at most major department stores

Cetaphil Daily Facial Moisturizer: www.cetaphil.com

Estee Lauder Verite Moisture Relief Crème and Soothing Spray Toner: www.esteelauder.com

Jurlique Ultra Sensitive Skincare: http://www.jurlique.com.au/

Biafine: www.biafine.com or (888) BIAFINE

Aquaphor Healing Ointment: www.eucerinus.com or your local pharmacy

DDF Organic Sunblock SPF 30: www.sephora.com or (877) 737-4672

Juvena Q10 Mask: www.sephora.com or (877) 737-4672

Osmotics Triceram-Ceramide Dominant Barrier Repair: www.sephora.com or (877) 737-4672

COMPLEMENTARY TREATMENTS FOR
THE SIDE EFFECTS OF RADIATION

Sesame oil: To avoid swollen mouth or red and blistered sores, gargle with sesame oil before and after each treatment.

Acupuncture: In addition to aiding the body to deal with all of the toxic effects of medication, acupuncture may also boost a woman's energy level.

Aromatherapy: Rosemary, bergamot, sandalwood, neroli, and melissa essential oils are of great benefit in relieving fatigue and lack of appetite following radiation. Camomile and fennel will combat nausea.

QUESTION 64. What questions should I ask my doctor about radiation therapy?

- Are you a radiation oncologist who specializes in breast cancer?
- How do I make sure that a facility is reliable?
- Why do I need radiation therapy?
- How is the radiation oncologist involved if therapists give the treatment?
- How will I evaluate the effectiveness of the treatments?
- Can I continue my usual work or exercise schedule?
- Can I miss a few treatments?
- Can I be treated elsewhere if I am traveling?
- What are the side effects of radiation therapy?
- Can the treated area be exposed to sunlight?
- How will radiation therapy affect my ability to conceive and bear children in the future?

HELPFUL HINT: *Coping with Skin Changes*

- Be extra kind to your skin in the treatment area. Do not use any soaps, lotions, deodorants, medicines, perfumes, cosmetics, talcum powder, or other substances without first speaking with your doctor.
- Wear loose-fitting clothes like soft cotton T-shirts.
- Avoid tight bra straps or underwire under the breast. Cushioning the area under the breast with a soft cotton cloth helps prevent irritation. You may feel more comfortable without a bra.
- Cornstarch can help keep the area cool and dry.
- Ask the nurse or physician for recommendations for soothing ointments if you need them.
- When you wash the area, use mild soap (without deodorant or perfumes) and lukewarm water.
- Do not scrub off the marks drawn on your skin by the therapist.
- Avoid extreme temperature—hot or cold.
- Protect the area from sun exposure.
- Do not use any forms of heat on treated area (hot water bottles, heating pads, etc.).
- Do not apply tape to the treated area.
- Do not shave your skin—use an electric shaver if you absolutely must, and only after you first consult with your doctor or nurse.
- Avoid exposure to the sun. Ask your doctor if you should use a PABA sunscreen.
- Keep your doctor informed of any skin changes—dryness, itching, or moist areas.
- Expose the treatment area to the air to aid the healing process.

8.

CHEMOTHERAPY

. . . .

QUESTION 65. What is chemotherapy?

Chemotherapy is the treatment of cancer with drugs that can destroy cancer cells, often called anticancer drugs. Chemotherapy can be used to help treat cancer, to control cancer, and to relieve symptoms that cancer may cause. Because some drugs work better together than alone, chemotherapy may consist of more than one drug. This is called combination chemotherapy.

Chemotherapy drugs are given as tablets or capsules or injected into a vein so as to enter your bloodstream. Tablets and capsules dissolve in your stomach, and the drug passes into your bloodstream. The drug is carried around your body in the bloodstream to reach the cancer cells. The drug gets into the cancer cells and may damage their genetic material (DNA). This may prevent the cancer cells from growing and dividing in an uncontrolled way.

Unfortunately, these drugs don't just affect cancer cells. They can damage any cells that are actively growing and dividing. For example, cells in the mouth, bone marrow, bowel, and hair roots are growing all the time. Chemotherapy may damage these normal cells, causing side effects such as sore mouth or hair loss. Normal cells recover quite quickly, so any damage they suffer is usually temporary. This is why most side effects go away once treatment is over.

Depending on the type of cancer and its stage of development, chemotherapy can be used:

- To cure cancer.
- To keep the cancer from spreading.
- To slow the cancer's growth.
- To kill cancer cells that may have spread to other parts of the body from the original tumor.
- To relieve symptoms that may be caused by the cancer.

QUESTION 66. How is chemotherapy given? How does my doctor determine the best treatment regimen?

Chemotherapy is usually given through intravenous (IV) injections, sometimes combined with pills. Treatment can be given at the hospital outpatient clinic, the doctor's office, or at home. It can last anywhere from 30 minutes to 4 hours. Many women find that bringing a friend for moral support or a CD or cassette of soothing music to treatment can be helpful during treatments. Treatment programs vary, but a typical course of chemotherapy runs 4 to 6 weeks, in 3- or 4-week cycles (a treatment period is followed by a recovery period, then another treatment period, etc.).

Patients who need many doses of IV chemotherapy often receive the drugs through a semipermanent catheter (a thin flexible tube) that allows the patient mobility and comfort. One end of the catheter is placed in a large vein in the chest. The other end is outside the body or attached to a small device just under the skin. Patients and their families are shown how to care for the catheter and keep it clean.

Chemotherapy regimens are tailored to the individual breast cancer patient. When planning a chemotherapy regimen, physicians and patients

consider the patient's age, her overall health, specific elements of her cancer (i.e., stage, grade, and other pathology prognostic factors), and past or
future treatments.

QUESTION 67. What are the most common side effects of chemotherapy?

Chemotherapy side effects will vary from woman to woman. The side effects that a woman will experience depend on several factors, including the
types of drugs used, their dosages, and the duration of treatment. Typical
side effects include: loss of appetite, nausea and vomiting, hair loss (alopecia), and mouth sores. Low blood cell counts (white and red blood cells)
and platelet counts are other possible side effects from chemotherapy. For
some women, medicines can be prescribed to help manage the side effects,
especially nausea and vomiting. Usually these side effects go away little by
little during the recovery period or after treatment stops.

Alopecia is a major concern for many patients. It is a temporary condition and may occur in some women because of weakened hair follicles.
Hair follicles consist of rapidly dividing cells, and chemotherapy indiscrim-
inately destroys fast-growing cells. This reaction causes hair to fall out at a
much faster rate than normal. For some women their hair will thin out,
while others may experience the loss of all body hair. Your hair may grow
back looking very different. Some women are shocked when they see that
their hair has changed color or their straight hair has turned curly or wavy.
Thin hair has been known to come back thick, and vice versa. Many people get what they started out with, but the key thing to remember is: *Your
hair will grow back.*

Patients may feel better if they decide how to handle hair loss before
starting treatment. There are several options available for women who lose
their hair during chemotherapy, including a variety of wigs and head wear.
The good news is, you will notice your hair growing back 4 to 6 weeks after your last treatment. Many people even see new hair growth before the
end of their treatment. The rate at which your hair grows back is related to
your age and your general health. If you are in pretty good shape, expect
the hair to grow about a half-inch a month.

Cancer patients who undergo chemotherapy should also be aware that chemotherapy drugs can cause infertility or induce premature menopause. The closer a woman is to menopause when she undergoes chemotherapy, the more likely she is to experience premature menopause. Women who are given chemotherapy often experience symptoms of menopause, such as hot flashes, vaginal dryness, and irregular menstrual cycles. These symptoms are not uncommon and can often be managed adequately.

> **Stacey Sforza,**
> *diagnosed age 39, stage IIIb*
>
> *"The oncology nurse advised me that my hair would fall out 17 days after my chemotherapy. I thought, 'Why didn't she pick a rounder number? 10 days? 15 days?' But 17 days later, I'm combing my hair, and whoop! there it went. I thought I would be devastated, but I surprised myself and took it pretty well. Hopefully, I can take the mastectomy just as well, but I don't think I will. I guess the difference is that I know my hair will grow back."*

Things to remember about the side effects of chemotherapy include:

- Many only happen on a few days of a treatment cycle, usually 24 to 72 hours after the chemotherapy infusion.
- Nearly all will go away a few months after completing treatment cycles.
- The doctor and nurses will work to prevent and reduce side effects.
- Most women maintain their jobs and daily activities during the weeks of adjuvant chemotherapy.

COMPLEMENTARY TREATMENT OPTIONS

Acupuncture: Acupuncture has been found to be very helpful prior to receiving chemotherapy to help avoid nausea.

American ginseng: For stress, American ginseng (*Panax quinquefolius*) can be taken as a supplement in the amount of 1 to 2 grams per day in capsule or tablet form or 3 to 5 milliliters of tincture 3 times per day.

Ginger: Many women use ginger as a supplement to ease nausea and vomiting following surgery and to ease nausea following chemotherapy. Some herbalists suggest the use of a tincture at 1.5 to 3 milliliters 3 times daily. Be sure to check with your doctor about using ginger, as there has been discussion that it might be contraindicated for some chemotherapy agents.

Imagery (visualization): The use of images in the mind's eye to overcome physical and mental ailments may be calming during chemotherapy treatment.

Lavender: This will often soothe insomnia and stress. Several drops of the oil can be added to a bath or diluted in vegetable oil for topical applications. The concentrated oil is not for internal use.

Meditation: Focusing your awareness on one thing, such as breath or a short phrase, will help to quiet the mind.

HELPFUL HINT: *Relieve Nausea, Sour Stomach, and Stressed-out Nerves*

- Try ginger ale mixed with 3 to 4 drops of bitters (available at the grocery store in the aisle with the soft drinks where the mixers are).
- Peppermints and sour lemon drops help combat nausea and the "metallic" taste many women experience in their mouths throughout chemotherapy.
- Ask your doctor about trying antiemetics that may help control nausea and vomiting. If a particular one isn't working well for you, try a different one, since different kinds work for different people.
- Eat foods that are friendly to your stomach, such as: toast, yogurt, ice chips, canned fruits, oatmeal, rice, and noodles.
- Consume foods and drinks at room temperature. Hot temperature may add to nausea. Speaking of hot—avoid foods that are spicy.
- Try breathing through your mouth when you feel nauseated.
- Remove dentures on days that you receive drug treatment.
- Eat before you get hungry. Once hunger sets in, chances are nausea will too.

HELPFUL HINT: *Wearing a Wig or Hat*

Like wearing pantyhose in the summer or stilettos a half size too small, wearing a wig can be downright uncomfortable. Wrap a long strip of quilter's cotton batting around your head before putting the wig on. It will help cushion against the scratchy inside of the wig, and allow some breathing room. The wig will fit much better, too, as it was meant to be worn over hair—not a bald head. The same advice works well with a variety of different hats.

QUESTION 68. What chemotherapy drugs are used to treat breast cancer?

Examples of chemotherapy combinations commonly used to treat early-diagnosed breast cancer include the following (the brand name of the drug is shown in parenthesis):

- *CMF:* cyclophosphamide (Cytoxan), methotrexate (Amethopterin, Mexate, Folex), and fluorouracil (Fluorouracil, 5-Fu, Adrucil)
- *CAF:* cyclophosphamide, doxorubicin (Adriamycin), and fluorouracil doxorubicin
- *AC:* doxorubicin, cyclophosphamide, and usually one of the taxanes (Taxol or Taxotere)
- *AT:* doxorubicin and cyclophosphamide with paclitaxel (Taxol), followed by CMF
- Cyclophosphamide, epirubicin (Ellence), and fluorouracil
- *FEC:* fluorouracil, epirubicin, and cyclophosphamide.
- Herceptin
- Taxol (or Taxotere)

Other chemotherapy drugs commonly used for treating women with metastatic or recurrent breast cancer include: docetaxel (Taxotere), vinorelbine

(Navelbine), gemcitabine (Gemzar), and capecitabine (Xeloda). See part 3 for a more complete list of cancer-related drugs.

HELPFUL HINT: *Dry Throat and Mouth Sores*

- Canned pineapple can sooth a sore mouth and help with a dry throat.
- All-natural mouthwash (preferably with tea tree oil, like Tom's of Maine) will help alleviate mouth sores (available at your health food store, Whole Foods, Fresh Fields, or Trader Joe's market).
- Mix 1 teaspoon of baking soda and ½ cup of warm water or club soda and rinse 4 times a day to alleviate mouth sores, reduce "cotton-mouth" feeling, and to fight bacteria.
- Carry a water bottle with you, so you can take frequent small sips of water.
- Suck on hard candy or popsicles. These tasty treats can help produce more saliva.

Complementary Treatment Options

- *Lactobacillus acidophilus and Lactobacillus bulgaricus:* Chewing 4 lacto-bacillus tablets, 3 times per day, may reduce soreness in some people with recurrent mouth ulcers.
- *Echinacea:* The well-documented antiviral, immune-enhancing, and wound-healing properties of echinacea make this herb a reasonable choice for mouth ulcers. Liquid echinacea in the amount of 4 milli-liters can be swished in the mouth for 2 to 3 minutes, then swallowed. This can be repeated 3 times per day. Tablets and capsules containing echinacea may also be helpful.

QUESTION 69. How will I know if my chemotherapy is working?

Your treatment team will use several methods to measure how well your treatments are working. You will have frequent physical examinations, blood tests, scans, and X rays. While tests and exams can tell a lot about how your therapy is working, side effects indicate very little. Side effects vary a great deal from person to person and from medication to medication. Having them or not having them is not a sign of whether the treatment is effective. Be sure to ask your doctor and/or nurse to discuss your test results with you and how these results indicate progress.

QUESTION 70. Can I still work while receiving chemotherapy?

First, you should consult with your doctor. Chemotherapy programs vary from person to person, and while some people report minimal side effects, you never know how your body will react until you've actually undergone treatment. If you choose to work while receiving chemotherapy, talk with your employer about adjusting your work schedule, or try working from home for a while. Federal and state laws sometimes require employers to allow a flexible work schedule to meet treatment needs. Your oncology social worker can assist you with this.

QUESTION 71. What will happen if I do not finish my recommended chemotherapy course? Will I be at risk for recurrence?

It is not uncommon for women to take a "time out" during the course of their chemotherapy treatment. In many situations, women are overwhelmed and distressed by the whole experience, and a week off should not disrupt the overall time schedule.

However, unless your doctor suggests otherwise, it's recommended to finish your chemotherapy course. Even when a patient completes an aggressive therapy treatment, there remains a possibility that some cancer cells

AMERICANS WITH DISABILITIES ACT (ADA)

. . . . . .

The ADA prohibits discrimination on the basis of disability in employment, state and local government, public accommodations, commercial facilities, transportation, and telecommunications. It also applies to the United States Congress. To be protected by the ADA, one must have a disability or have a relationship or association with an individual with a disability. An individual with a disability is defined by the ADA as a person who has a physical or mental impairment that substantially limits one or more major life activities, a person who has a history or record of such an impairment, or a person who is perceived by others as having such an impairment. The ADA does not specifically name all of the impairments that are covered.

Discrimination is not only morally wrong but it also undermines critical public health efforts to fight the breast cancer epidemic. The fear of discrimination can lead to disastrous delays in the treatment of individual patients, and deters women from accessing the health care system. Now more than ever people living with breast cancer need unencumbered access to health care. Treatment options have dramatically improved the health and prolonged the lives of many women with breast cancer. Any barrier to seeking treatment, such as discrimination by a physician or employer, is unacceptable and can truly be a matter of life and death.

To obtain answers to general and technical questions about the ADA, call: 800-514-0301 (voice), 800-514-0383 (TTY), or visit www.usdoj.gov/crt/ada/adahom1.htm (the U.S. Department of Justice website).

The Americans with Disabilities Act: Protection for Cancer Patients against Employment Discrimination (4585, 1993)

This publication defines the ADA law by describing the employment rights of the cancer patient. Call the American Cancer Society, (800) ACS-2345, or your local chapter for a free copy.

survived. These cells can eventually repopulate and grow into a focus of recurrent disease. Follow-up examinations are scheduled posttreatment to screen for such recurrences. Screening includes monthly self-examinations by the patient, periodic history and physical examinations by a physician, and periodic blood and X-ray tests.

If you are undergoing cancer treatment, expect to experience fatigue. If you need to take time off from work, don't be shy about asking your employer. Whether you choose to work part- or full-time or have a flexible schedule (and a kind employer), try to arrive at work early. Your energy levels will drop throughout the day, and you'll be perkiest in the morning. Take a short walk after about an hour at work: the perfect excuse to grab a cup of morning tea. After about three hours, eat a small meal with protein. Then shut your eyes, space out, and concentrate on absolutely nothing for a few minutes. These minibreaks will help keep you energized throughout the day. After work, have a small snack and try to sit again for a short time. You'll be better prepared to take advantage of the moments when you feel okay and will be more productive. *Remember that you are not alone.* Studies have shown that general fatigue, including fatigue caused by anemia, affects more than three-quarters of patients undergoing cancer treatment.

Complementary Options

Physical exercise: Something as simple and inexpensive as power walking regularly may lead to a better quality of life in terms of energy level and self-esteem.

Vitamin B_{12}: B_{12} deficiency can contribute to fatigue, and B_{12} is easy to supplement through your diet. It is found in all foods of animal origin, including dairy, eggs, meat and poultry, and fish.

Acupuncture: Chronic fatigue, insomnia, problems concentrating, and poor stamina can be reduced with the help of acupuncture.

QUESTION 72. What questions should I ask my doctor about chemotherapy?

- Should I start chemotherapy before surgery?
- Why do I need chemotherapy? What criteria were used to determine this for me?
- What are the risks of chemotherapy?

- Are there any other possible treatment methods?
- Are there any clinical trials for my type and stage of cancer?
- How many treatments will I be given and how often?
- What drug(s) will I be taking? How will they be given?
- Where will I receive my treatment?
- How long will each treatment last?
- What are the possible side effects of the chemotherapy? What can I do to relieve the side effects?
- Clinical trials are a valuable resource that should be considered. What clinical trials are available for me, and how do I decide if I should participate in one?

HELPFUL HINT: *How to Handle Loss of Appetite*

- A diet high in vitamins and protein is very important.
- Eat 6 to 7 small meals instead of 3 large meals.
- Let others cook for you.
- Consult your doctor about taking nutritional supplements to increase intake.
- Keep your doctor informed of any problems with eating.

Complementary Options

- *Acupuncture:* Can increase appetite, which might be useful after chemotherapy.
- *Horehound* (Marrubium vulgare): The major active element is marrubiin; along with some of the oils found in the herb, it is believed to be responsible for expectorant action. In addition, marrubiin is an herbal bitter that increases the flow of saliva and gastric juice, thereby stimulating the appetite.
- *St. John's wort* is a wild-growing herb with yellow flowers. Today, the herb is a popular treatment for mild to moderate depression, and many other conditions, including loss of appetite. If you are currently taking antidepressants, it is important to consult your doctor before taking St. John's wort.

9.

HORMONAL THERAPY

· ·

QUESTION 73. My doctor has
recommended
hormonal therapy.
What does this mean?

Hormonal therapy is used to prevent the growth, spread, or recurrence of breast cancer. If lab tests show that your tumor depends on your natural hormones to grow, it will be described as estrogen-positive or progesterone-positive in the lab report. This means that any remaining cancer cells may continue to grow when these hormones are present in your body. Hormonal therapy can block your body's natural hormones from reaching any remaining cancer cells. One of the most common drugs used for hormonal therapy for breast cancer is tamoxifen.

QUESTION 74. What is tamoxifen and how does it work?

Tamoxifen is a selective estrogen receptor modulator (SERM) that is an antiestrogen drug. This means that it reduces or stops the action of the female hormone estrogen. Many breast cancers rely on supplies of sex hormones, particularly estrogen, to grow. Cancers with estrogen receptors on the surface of their cells are called *estrogen receptor–positive* (ER-positive). When the sex hormones come into contact with the receptors, they activate the cancer cells to divide, and the tumor grows. Tamoxifen prevents the estrogen from reaching the cancer cells, so they either grow more slowly or stop growing altogether. It is usually prescribed as a single daily dose, and this should be taken at the same time each day. Some women prefer to take it with food, as it may cause feelings of temporary sickness and leave a metallic taste in your mouth.

Tamoxifen was developed over 20 years ago and is now widely used to treat breast cancer in women whose tumors are hormone receptor–positive. Trials are under way to decide exactly how long tamoxifen should be taken after surgery breast cancer. It is commonly prescribed for five years.

QUESTION 75. What are the side effects of tamoxifen?

Side effects are more common in premenopausal women, who may develop menopausal side effects as a result of a reduced level of estrogen. However, for most women the benefits of tamoxifen far outweigh the risks.

- *Common side effects* include mild nausea, hot flashes, and sweats (particularly at night).
- *Less common side effects* are depression, tiredness, and dizziness.
- *Rare side effects* are allergic reactions (may include skin rashes), temporary thinning of the hair, headaches, flaking fingernails (after several years of treatment), thrombosis (blood clots; pain, warmth, swelling,

or tenderness in an arm or leg or any chest pain must be reported to your doctor immediately), visual problems (blurred/reduced vision is rare but should be reported to your doctor), and voice changes have been reported by some women. Studies have also shown that women who take high doses of tamoxifen over a long period of time may have an increased risk of developing endometrial cancer.

• *The most serious side effects* include uterine cancer, blood clots in the lungs and large blood vessels, and stroke. Although these risks are "rare," they are real—and they are most likely to happen in women over 50, the women at greatest risk for breast cancer and therefore most likely to take tamoxifen as a preventive measure. In addition, any woman with a uterus who takes tamoxifen should be monitored annually with an endometrial biopsy, a painful and expensive procedure.

HELPFUL HINT: *Managing Hot Flashes*

"Soy works for some women. Even though some people are nervous about soy, there is one study of soy protein in conjunction with tamoxifen in rats that shows they work together; they don't counteract each other. Black cohosh actually doesn't completely get rid of hot flashes, but it does reduce them. Remifemin is a good way to get black cohosh. If they're worse than that, some of the antidepressants like Effexor (venlafaxine) have been shown to reduce hot flashes in some women."

Susan Love, M.D., *adjunct professor of surgery at UCLA and medical director of the Susan Love, M.D., Breast Cancer Foundation (at the 2001 San Antonio Breast Cancer Symposium)*

QUESTION 76. What questions should I ask my doctor about hormone therapy?

• What benefit might I get from hormonal therapy?
• What drug will I be taking? How will I know that it is working?

Amy Spiegel,
diagnosed age 41, stage I

"I started tamoxifen on September 29, 2001, and was in great fear of the side effects but wanted to reduce my risk as much as possible. So far, the side effect that caused the most trouble for me was extremely intense, severe, and hourly hot flashes. Drugs didn't help, but acupuncture eliminated them completely. I was extremely fearful of weight gain. However, I am active, and I started a weight management class, and I am controlling my weight."

- What are the side effects and how do I manage them?
- How long will I be on hormonal therapy?
- Will I need follow-up care?
- What if I don't have hormonal therapy?
- Can I get pregnant while taking tamoxifen?
- What is the latest research data on the safety of tamoxifen?
- What is the latest research data on how long to take tamoxifen?
- Are there drugs other than tamoxifen for hormonal therapy?

10.

COMPLEMENTARY &
ALTERNATIVE THERAPIES

. . . .

If you've never thought about or tried complementary therapies, like massage therapy, acupuncture, yoga, or relaxation techniques, to treat breast cancer, you may want to open your mind up to the possibility. Complementary therapies may bring some much-needed comfort. Besides, it's always wise to educate yourself with all of your health choices.

The decision to use complementary/alternative medicine is an important one. Before selecting a complementary or alternative therapy, it is essential to consider:

- The safety and effectiveness of the therapy or treatment.
- The expertise and qualifications of the health care practitioner.
- The quality of the service delivery.

It is imperative to communicate with your doctors about any complementary therapies you might be undergoing. Some therapies may interact negatively with your prescribed treatment plan. For example, taking vitamin C in tablet form during chemotherapy with Adriamycin will prevent the chemotherapy from working properly. Taking shark cartilage directly before or after surgery will prevent your wound from healing. These issues should be considered when selecting *any* practitioner or therapy.

Various integrative approaches to medicine, such as traditional Chinese medicine, herbal therapies, and alternative treatments, are outlined and discussed extensively in part 2.

QUESTION 77. What are alternative/complementary therapies and treatments?

The term "complementary and alternative medicine" (CAM) covers a broad range of healing philosophies, approaches, and therapies. Many therapies are dubbed "holistic," which typically means that the health care practitioner treats the whole person, including physical, mental, emotional, and spiritual aspects. Generally, CAM includes treatments and health care practices not widely taught in medical schools, not generally used in hospitals, and not usually reimbursed by medical insurance companies. People use these treatments and therapies in a variety of ways. Therapies are used alone (often referred to as alternative), in combination with other alternative therapies, or in addition to conventional therapies (often referred to as complementary).

QUESTION 78. How do complementary/ alternative treatments differ from standard medical treatments?

Some CAM approaches are consistent with physiological principles of Western medicine, while others represent healing systems with different origins. While some therapies are far outside the realm of accepted Western medical theory and practice, others are becoming more widely accepted and established in mainstream medicine.

QUESTION 79. How can I find out about *safe* and *effective* CAM treatments?

Specific information about an alternative or complementary therapy's safety and effectiveness is usually less readily available than information about conventional medical treatments. You may want to ask a health care practitioner, whether a physician or CAM practitioner, about the safety and effectiveness of the therapy or treatment he or she is recommending. Health care providers are becoming more and more familiar with CAM treatments, but if unable to answer your questions, they may be able to refer you to someone more CAM-savvy. Medical libraries, public libraries, and popular bookstores are also good places to find information about particular complementary and alternative medical practices. Be sure to inform your practitioner about any CAM treatments you may already be receiving, as this information may be crucial in determining the safety and effectiveness of your entire treatment plan.

QUESTION 80. How can I check on the qualifications of the people providing alternative methods of treatment?

According to Beverly Burns, director of the Charlotte Maxwell Complementary Clinic in Oakland, California, currently there are no standardized systems in place to check the qualifications of CAM providers. "This is a big issue, because many organizations are concerned about liability and so they will not endorse or deny ["un-endorse"] anyone. We [CMCC] are trying to get a grant at UCSF to work on this, but so far [with] no success," says Burns. While there is no formal system in place when looking for an alternative health practitioner, it is advisable to do your homework before making a medical commitment. Word-of-mouth referrals have always worked wonders for me, personally. You can also consult your local grass-roots women's organizations or post an inquiry on your local online bulletin board. Here in San Francisco, I've received countless successful referrals on www.craigslist.com. The site includes listings for many cities across the country. Peer referrals are invaluable when you want an unbiased opinion. You can also consider the person's professional training and ask for references.

QUESTION 81. What questions should I ask my doctor about CAM?

- Ask your health care practitioner, whether a physician or a practitioner of complementary and alternative health care, about the safety and effectiveness of the therapy or treatment he or she uses.
- What claims are made for the treatment? (Does it claim to cure cancer? To enable the conventional treatment to work better? To relieve symptoms or side effects?)
- What are the credentials of the people or organizations supporting the treatment?
- Are they recognized experts in cancer treatment?
- Have their findings been published in trustworthy medical journals?
- How is the method promoted? Is it promoted only in the mass media? Is it mentioned in scientific journals?
- Ask the practitioner how many patients he or she typically sees in a day or week, and how much time the practitioner spends with the patient. Take notice of the conditions of the office or clinic.
- What are the costs of the therapy? Ask your practitioner and your health insurer which treatments or therapies are reimbursable.
- Is the method widely available for use within the health care community, or is it controlled, with limited access to its use?
- Does the method require that you forego conventional therapy? If so, will doing so affect any chances for cure?
- Is the cancer stage likely to advance during the delay?

11.

CLINICAL TRIALS

. . . .

QUESTION 82. What are clinical trials?

Clinical trials are also called *medical research* and *research studies*. A clinical trial is a carefully designed research study that usually involves comparing one treatment with another. Clinical trials are used to determine whether new drugs or treatments are both safe and effective. There are also clinical trials that examine tumor markers or deal with quality-of-life and exercise issues.

As a volunteer in a clinical trial, you are participating in the development of important medical therapies. People volunteer to participate in a clinical trial for many reasons. You may get involved in a trial because you simply want to help in the advancement of science. You may join a clinical trial hoping to improve the medical care you receive. If you do not have health insurance, clinical trials are a way to receive study-related medical care. Patients must meet very strict eligibility criteria in order to participate in a clinical trial.

Clinical trials of experimental drugs proceed through four phases:

- **Phase 1:** Researchers test a new drug or treatment in a small group of people (20 to 80) for the first time to evaluate its safety, determine a safe dosage range, and identify side effects.

- **Phase 2:** The study drug or treatment is given to a larger group of people (100 to 300) to see if it is effective and to further evaluate its safety.
- **Phase 3:** The study drug or treatment is given to large groups of people (1,000 to 3,000) to confirm its effectiveness, monitor side effects, compare it to commonly used treatments, and collect information that will allow the drug or treatment to be used safely.
- **Phase 4:** Studies are done after the drug or treatment has been marketed. These studies continue testing the study drug or treatment to collect information about their effect in various populations and any side effects associated with long-term use.

Clinical trials can be either "randomized" or "double-blinded." Randomized means to randomly assign subjects to groups after they have been identified and enrolled into the study. The assignment to a group is not known prior to the time the assignment is made. A double-blinded trial is a clinical trial in which neither the medical staff nor the person knows which of several possible therapies the person is receiving.

QUESTION 83. How are clinical trials conducted? How are patients protected?

The clinical trial process depends on the kind of trial you participate in. For all types of trials, you will work with a research team. The team will include doctors and nurses as well as social workers and other health care professionals. They will check your health at the beginning of the trial, give you specific instructions for participating, monitor your health to determine the safety and effectiveness of their treatment, and stay in touch with you after the study.

Some clinical trials involve more tests and doctor visits than you would typically undergo for your condition. Your participation will be most successful if you follow the protocol carefully and stay in contact with the research staff. A protocol describes what types of people may participate in the trial; the schedule of tests, procedures, medications, and dosages; and the length of the study.

CLINICAL TRIALS:
WEIGHING THE PROS AND CONS

· · · · · ·

While a clinical trial is a good choice for some people, this treatment option has both possible benefits and drawbacks. Here are some factors to consider. You may want to discuss them with your doctor and the people close to you.

Possible Benefits

- Clinical trials offer high-quality cancer care. If you are in a study and do not receive the new treatment being tested, you will receive the best standard treatment. This may be as good as, or better than, the new approach.
- If a new treatment approach is proven to work and you are taking it, you may be among the first to benefit.
- By looking at the pros and cons of clinical trials and your other treatment choices, you are taking an active role in a decision that affects your life.
- You have the chance to help others and improve cancer treatment.

Possible Drawbacks

- New treatments under study are not always better than standard care. They may have side effects that doctors do not expect or that are worse than those of standard treatment.
- Even if a new treatment has benefits, it may not work for you. Even standard treatments that have proven effective for many people do not help everyone.
- If you receive standard treatment instead of the new treatment being tested, it may not be as effective as the new approach.
- Health insurance and managed care providers do not always cover all patient care costs in a study. What they cover varies by plan and by study. To find out in advance what costs are likely to be paid in your case, talk to a doctor, nurse, or social worker from the study.

The government has strict guidelines to protect people who choose to participate in clinical trials. Every clinical trial in the United States must be approved and monitored by an institutional review board (IRB), which is an independent committee of physicians, statisticians, community advocates, and others that ensures that the clinical trial is ethical, that the rights of study participants are protected, and that the risks are as low as possible and are worth any potential benefits.

QUESTION 84. What is informed consent?

Informed consent is a process in which you learn the key facts about a research study before you decide whether or not to participate. In addition to your talking about these facts with the research doctor or nurse, they will be included in a written consent form that you can take home to read and discuss. If English is not your first language, you can ask for the consent documents in languages other than English. The consent form includes what type of medical care or condition is being researched, how long the study will last, possible risks and benefits, and the tests you may have. If you decide to join the clinical trial, be sure to ask for a copy of the informed consent documents so you can review them at any time. Since joining a clinical trial is an important decision, you should ask the research team any questions you may have about the study and the consent forms before you make a decision. You may also ask the research team any questions you have at any time during the study. You can change your mind and withdraw from the study at any time before or during the study.

QUESTION 85. What is the Breast Cancer Prevention Trial?

The Breast Cancer Prevention Trial (BCPT) was a clinical trial funded by the National Cancer Institute and conducted by the National Surgical Adjuvant Breast and Bowel Project (NSABP). The BCPT was designed to see whether tamoxifen (see chapter 9) could prevent breast cancer in women who are at an increased risk of developing this disease. The study began recruiting participants in April 1992 and closed enrollment in September 1997. This study involved 13,388 premenopausal and postmenopausal women at more than 300 centers across the United States and Canada and is one of the largest breast cancer prevention studies to date.

Results of the BCPT were reported in the September 16, 1998, issue of the *Journal of the National Cancer Institute.*

QUESTION 86. What is a bone marrow transplant (BMT)?

High-level chemotherapy severely damages the bone marrow of breast cancer patients, thereby seriously depleting the immune system. In order for some patients to benefit from this aggressive treatment, they may need to undergo a *bone marrow transplant.* After chemotherapy treatment, a patient will receive matching donor tissue, or their own tissue that was harvested prior to treatment (called *autologous BMT*), to replenish their damaged bone marrow with healthy tissue.

Bone marrow is a spongy tissue found inside the bones. The bone marrow in the breastbone, skull, hips, ribs, and spine contains stem cells that produce the body's blood cells. These blood cells include white blood cells (leukocytes), which fight infection; red blood cells (erythrocytes), which carry oxygen to and remove waste products from organs and tissues; and platelets, which enable the blood to clot.

A BMT is a physically, emotionally, and psychologically taxing procedure for both the patient and family. The patient must stay in the hospital for several weeks, away from home, family, and work. The hospital room must be kept sterile. Visitors must take strict precautions, as they might carry a simple infection that could devastate a patient with a damaged immune system. Compared with those receiving standard chemotherapy, these patients experience higher risks of a life-threatening infection and increased occurrences of nausea, mouth sores, pain (fever), and generalized discomfort. At this point, BMTs are being performed only as part of clinical trials and used for breast cancer treatment only in rare situations.

QUESTION 87.   Who is a candidate for a bone marrow transplant?

Patients are considered on a case-by-case basis, and the disease criteria for eligibility for a bone marrow/stem cell transplant includes:

• Non-Hodgkin's lymphoma.
• Hodgkin's disease.
• Acute myeloid leukemia.
• Chronic myeloid leukemia.
• Multiple myeloma.
• Breast cancer.
• Ovarian cancer.
• Germ cell tumors.

Patients with any of these listed diseases or conditions must also be between 18 and 70 years of age, have no significant heart, lung, kidney, or liver diseases, and be able to understand the risks and benefits of the procedure.

QUESTION 88.   How can I obtain a list of clinical trials for breast cancer?

Breast cancer patients and their family members are frequently in search of information about the latest drugs being researched to treat the patient's cancer. That drug research is being conducted through the clinical trials process. Some of the locations that conduct breast cancer clinical trials or list breast cancer trials that are being conducted are as follows.

The CenterWatch Clinical Trials Listing Service
www.centerwatch.com
This clinical trials listing service offers information on over 40,000+ clinical trials actively seeking study volunteers.

The Cancer Information Service

http://cis.nci.nih.gov

(800) 4-CANCER

The Cancer Information Service (CIS), a national information and education network, is a free public service of the National Cancer Institute (NCI). If you go to their website, click on "Other Cancer Resources," and then "Clinical Trials."

The National Cancer Institute (NCI)

http://cancernet.nci.nih.gov

(800) 422-6237

The NCI's PDQ database contains close to 2,000 cancer clinical trials. The phone service provides information about cancer clinical trials as well as general information about cancer treatment, diagnosis, and screening.

U.S. National Institutes of Health

http://clinicaltrials.gov/ct/gui

(888) 346-3656

The NIH, through its National Library of Medicine, has developed this website to provide patients, family members, and members of the public with current information about clinical research studies. Check often for regular updates.

U.S. Food and Drug Association (FDA)

www.fda.gov/oashi/cancer/trials.html

(301) 827-4460 (Office of Special Health Issues)

The FDA lists clinical trials by specific tumor type.

If you live outside of the United States:

International Union Against Cancer (UICC)

3, rue du Conseil General

1205 Geneva

Switzerland

http://www.uicc.org

41 22 809 18 11

The International Union Against Cancer (UICC) consists of international cancer-related organizations devoted to the worldwide fight against cancer. UICC membership includes research facilities and treatment centers and, in some countries, ministries of health. Other members include volunteer cancer leagues, associations, and societies. These organizations serve as resources for the public and may have helpful information about cancer, treatment centers, and research studies.

The European Organization for Research and Treatment of Cancer (EORTC)
Avenue Mounier, 83
B1200 Brussels
Belgium
http://www.eortc.be
32 (2) 774 16 11

The EORTC maintains information about clinical trials being conducted in European countries.

QUESTION 89. What questions should I ask about clinical trials?

- What is the purpose of the study? In what phase is this study?
- Why do researchers believe the new treatment may be effective? Has it been tested before?
- How are the study data and patient safety being checked?
- When and where will the study results go?
- What are the possible short- and long-term risks, side effects, and benefits to me?
- What is involved in terms of tests, treatments, and additional time commitments?
- Where will my treatment take place? Will I have to be in the hospital? If so, for how long?
- Can you put me in touch with other people who are in this study?
- What results can be reasonably expected in my particular case?
- What are the currently accepted treatments and how do they compare to the trial?

- What would my financial commitment be, and how can I cope with it? Who can help answer any questions from my insurance company or managed-care plan?
- Will I need to be available for follow-up testing indefinitely?
- If I participate in a double-blinded study, when will I know if I'm receiving chemo dose X versus chemo dose Y?

12.

METASTASIS

. . . .

QUESTION 90. What is metastatic cancer?

When an invasive breast cancer tumor grows, it has the ability to shed cancerous cells that metastasize (or spread) to other parts of the body through the bloodstream and the lymph system. When the cancer spreads, it can form new tumors in other parts of the body. These spreading tumors are called metastases. Metastatic breast cancer is the most advanced stage (stage IV) of breast cancer. The symptoms of metastasis depend on the site of spread.

General Symptoms
- Chronic localized bone pain (possible indication of bone metastases).
- An enlarged liver found during a physical exam may indicate liver metastases.
- Lung metastases are usually found on a chest X ray or lung scan.
- Shortness of breath (possible indication of lung metastases).
- Lack of appetite (possible indication of liver metastases).
- Weight loss (possible indication of liver metastases).
- Neurological pain or weakness, headaches (possible indications of neurological metastases).

QUESTION 91.

Where does breast cancer commonly metastasize?

A site for metastatic cancer must have a blood supply and an environment where it can grow. When the cancer spreads, it can form new tumors in other parts of the body. Metastases can be found in the liver, lungs, brain, and the bones of the pelvis, spine, legs, ribs, and skull. Your doctor may diagnose metastatic breast cancer by using a number of diagnostic tests in combination with your medical history and a physical exam. Metastases, if they are going to occur, do so most often within the first 3 years after initial diagnosis for breast cancer. Sometimes they are found at the same time as the primary breast lump if the cancer has been growing for some time.

> **Joanne Bussiere,**
> *diagnosed age 34, stage I*
>
> *"When I was first diagnosed with breast cancer I did not know much about metastasis. I thought I'd have the lumpectomy and radiation (and chemotherapy) and that would be it, no big deal. Unfortunately, metastasis is a concern. Breast cancer can find its way to one's lungs, liver, bones, or brain. The most important thing here is to stay aware of your body and 'symptoms of mets' without becoming overcome by its possibility. Focus on life in a quality way."*

QUESTION 92. I have been diagnosed with a metastasis. What are my treatment options?

The treatment for breast cancer depends on the size of the tumor and how much it has spread. In most cases, surgery is done to remove the tumor and all or part of the breast and the axillary lymph nodes, which helps the staging of the disease. The treatments for metastatic breast cancer include radiation, chemotherapy, and hormone therapies. You may have just one type of treatment or a combination of treatments. These treatments are not expected to cure metastatic cancer, but they do help to slow down growth of the tumor and decrease its size so that the symptoms decrease. In some cases, remission is possible.

QUESTION 93. I have metastatic breast cancer that has spread to my bones. What are my available treatment options?

While bone metastases can be difficult to live with, there are many treatment options available for alleviating pain and treating the cancer itself. These treatments include:

For local recurrence
- Surgery, usually mastectomy.
- Radiation.
- Chemotherapy.
- Hormone therapy.
- Regional recurrence.
- Surgery (chest wall).
- Radiation.
- Chemotherapy.
- Hormone therapy.

For distant recurrence
- Surgery (if an isolated tumor).
- Radiation.
- Hormone therapy.
- High-dose chemotherapy.
- Bone marrow/stem cell transplant.
- Clinical trials.

Aredia (pamidronate disodium): Aredia is prescribed for women to help reduce further bone breakdown, relieve pain, and minimize fractures. Aredia is not an anticancer drug and has no effect on the cancer cells themselves. It works by blocking the breakdown of bone from the cancer and reducing complications from the bone metastases. Aredia is given intravenously as an outpatient procedure every 4 weeks.

Chemotherapy: These days, there are specific chemotherapy drugs for metastasis. Chemotherapy treatment options are influenced by the drugs the patient has previously been given, the potential for side effects (such as low white blood cell count), age, other medical conditions, and the extent of disease. In addition, the administration schedule required can also be an important factor. If you have to choose between a treatment that would require a visit to your oncologist once a week versus once every 3 weeks, you might prefer going to the doctor less often.

Radiation therapy: Many women receive adjuvant radiation therapy at the site of their bone metastases to relieve pain. The relief generated by radiation tends not to last as long but can be effective for some people.

Hormone therapy: Hormone therapy is very effective in controlling the cancer that has spread to the bones and in relieving any symptoms, and no other therapy may be needed if that is the only area of metastasis. Many women who are ER-positive and have bone metastasis are given an aromatase inhibitor, like Arimidex or Femara, which can stabilize and even fight the disease in the bone.

Quadramet: Quadramet alleviates bone pain and targets osteoblastic lesions. An injection of Quadramet, administered by a certified nuclear medicine technologist, can relieve bone pain for weeks or months.

Pain medication: You will probably take medication to relieve your pain. Even severe pain can be controlled by a combination of medicines, which usually include narcotics. People who are placed on narcotics to control pain do not become drug addicts. As radiation or chemotherapy treatment relieves the pain, the need for pain medication will gradually disappear.

QUESTION 94. How can I reduce my chance of getting an infection?

Particular genetic changes in the breast cancer may make it more prone to spread. There are several factors that contribute to metastasis, but the strength of the person's immune system is crucial, and infection should be avoided.

- Stay away from people who have infections, such as a cold or the flu.
- Stay away from people who have open sores, such as cold sores.
- Be careful about personal hygiene, especially after using the bathroom.
- Take good care of your skin to help prevent cracks and cuts.
- Have dental work done only when your doctor or oncologist says your white blood cell count is in the acceptable range.
- Give up gardening (just for a while!) in order to avoid soil contaminants.
- Delegate the tasks of cleaning the cat's litter pan or the bird cage and walking the dog to someone else so that you have no contact with pets' leavings.
- Avoid raw or improperly prepared food, which may harbor infectious bacteria. Careful food handling, storage, preparation, cooking, and serving can help you avoid infection from food sources and preparation utensils.

QUESTION 95. What questions should I ask my doctor about metastasis?

- Where has my breast cancer metastasized?
- How many metastatic sites are there?
- What is my estrogen and progesterone receptor status?
- What is my HER2/neu status?
- What treatment do you recommend?
- What other treatment options are available if the first one doesn't work?
- How can I manage pain systems?
- How can I improve my overall quality of life?
- What is my estimated prognosis?

13.

PROGNOSIS & RECURRENCE

. . . .

Prognosis cannot be completely predicted. There are some general guidelines as to the potential biological behavior of a breast carcinoma. In general, a better prognosis will accompany cancers that are:

- Less than 2 centimeters in size.
- Without axillary (underarm) lymph node involvement.
- Noninvasive ductal carcinoma and LCIS.
- ER- and PR-positive.
- Without aneuploidy.

QUESTION 96. What are the survival statistics for breast cancer?

Many factors influence breast cancer survival. The clinical stage of breast cancer is the best indicator for prognosis (probable outcome), in addition to some other factors. It is important to remember, as with any statistical data, that the figures apply to populations of individuals and therefore cannot be

Joanne Bussiere,
diagnosed age 34, stage I

"Prognosis is a term that is ultimately hard to tap into. The truth is that no one can say for sure how much time any of us have. I asked for a prognosis after being told of my metastasis. My doctor said she did not like to answer that because each case is different. I wanted a definite answer, but now I truly understand that no one can predict the future. New treatments, a person's attitude, and what is not ours to control all factor into this; what is most important is to truly live while we are alive."

used to tell the exact outcome for a given individual in advance. Five-year survival rates for individuals with breast cancer who receive appropriate treatment are approximately:

- 95 percent for stage 0.
- 88 percent for stage I.
- 66 percent for stage II.
- 36 percent for stage III.
- 7 percent for stage IV.

Axillary (underarm) lymph nodes are the main passageway that breast cancer cells use to reach the rest of the body. How they play into the scenario strongly affects the prognosis. Chemotherapy and hormone therapy can improve prognosis in all patients and increase the likelihood of cure in patients with stage I, II, and III disease.

Based on most recent data, relative survival rates for women diagnosed with breast cancer are:

- 85 percent at 5 years after diagnosis.
- 76 percent after 10 years.
- 58 percent after 15 years.
- 53 percent after 20 years.

The 5-year relative survival rate for breast cancer increases with age at diagnosis until age 75:

- 82 percent for women under 45.
- 86 percent for women 45 to 54.
- 87 percent for women 55 to 64.
- 88 percent for women 65 to 74.
- 84 percent for women 75 and older.

QUESTION 97.   What are the symptoms and types of a breast cancer recurrence?

Occasionally breast cancer can return after primary treatment. Recurrences occur because cells were left behind in the breast, lymph nodes, or chest wall (a local recurrence) or cells got into the blood vessels and traveled to other parts of the body such as bones, liver, or lungs (a systemic recurrence). The word for the movement of cancer cells is "metastasize," and the new growths in other organs are called "metastases." Often, a diagnosis of recurrent cancer is more devastating or psychologically difficult for a woman than her initial breast cancer diagnosis. Women who have recurrent breast cancer are encouraged to discuss their feelings with a counselor or therapist and consider joining a support group. There are three types of recurrent breast cancer.

Local recurrence: Cancerous tumor cells remain in the original site and, over time, grow back. Most physicians do not consider local breast cancer recurrence to be the spread of breast cancer but a failure of the primary treatment. Even after mastectomy, portions of the breast skin and fat remain, and local recurrence is possible but uncommon.

Regional recurrence: This is more serious than local recurrence, because it usually indicates that the cancer has spread past the breast and the axillary (underarm) lymph nodes. Regional breast cancer recurrences can occur in the pectoral (chest) muscles, in the internal mammary lymph nodes, under the breastbone and between the ribs, in the supraclavicular nodes (above the collarbone), and in the nodes surrounding the neck.

Distant recurrence: A distant breast cancer recurrence, also known as a metastasis, is the most precarious type of recurrence. Once out of the breast, cancer usually spreads first to the axillary (underarm) lymph nodes. In 25 percent of distant recurrences, breast cancer spreads from the lymph nodes to bone. Other sites breast cancer may spread to include the bone marrow, lungs, liver, brain, and other organs.

Most systemic recurrences cause symptoms. The symptoms depend on which organ is affected. For example, breast cancer that has traveled to the bones will often cause pain. It is often difficult for a patient who has recently been diagnosed to know which symptoms might be indicative of recurrent disease and which symptoms are simply normal aches and pains. It takes time for a woman to start trusting her body again after a diagnosis of breast cancer. In general, symptoms of recurrence are more persistent than normal aches and pains and become progressively more severe. If you are worried about a new symptom, especially if it is persistent or getting worse, you should see your doctor. Not all new symptoms mean a recurrence of breast cancer, but your doctor should evaluate them and arrive at a diagnosis.

QUESTION 98. Why and where does breast cancer commonly recur?

Breast cancer can recur either locally, regionally, or at distant sites. *Local recurrence* in the breast most often occurs after breast-conserving treatment but can do so after mastectomy in the form of recurrence in the wound. *Regional recurrence* refers to the detection of breast cancer either in the axillary nodes, in internal mammary nodes, or in the supraclavicular nodes. *Distant recurrence* is when tumor appears elsewhere in the body, most commonly in the lungs, bones, and liver.

QUESTION 99. Is it possible to maintain a sense of humor throughout all of this?

Not only is it possible, it is necessary! Breast cancer is a life-threatening disease, which challenges the body and spirit. It tries to belittle its victim and can make you question who you are. Fear, sadness, and despondency often produce negative outcomes while a humorous outlook can help in the healing process. Although breast cancer is no laughing matter, the role of humor and laughter in the healing process for breast cancer is rarely discussed or prescribed by physicians. If you let it, breast cancer can take the life out of your life. Celebrate life—a little laughter can go a long way.

QUESTION 100.   So, I've made it this far. Where do I go now for more information?

The good news is that you now have basic working knowledge of the wide world of breast cancer. The less-than-stellar news is that you can't stop your quest for information here. Consider your diagnosis an ongoing research project, because the more you know, the better equipped you will be to make smart decisions—the best decisions for *you*. Be fearless in asking your doctors, nurses, and medical treatment team members for information. They may have fancy diplomas on their office walls, and lack compassion from time to time, but the bottom line is that you have a right to know anything your heart desires about your health, your body, and your specific diagnosis. If, at first, you have difficulty asking questions or getting answers, don't give up. Have someone intervene on your behalf to obtain answers, medical records, and general explanations. Your energy may not be operating at full throttle, and this is a simple solution to an often stressful task.

Another helpful hint is to join a support group. There is nothing quite like womanly bonds, and when you throw a terrifying disease into the scenario, the strength and invaluable "been there" advice provided from such groups is incredible. The fact is that breast cancer is an ongoing battle, and it's easier to face adversity when you have an army of strength and support behind you. You may be the toughest gal in the world, but now is not the time to keep a stiff upper lip, or, as the adage goes, "Grin and bear it."

Don't be afraid to ask for help. Read everything you can get your hands on. There are constant changes in the world of breast cancer, and being on top of your game is key to staying informed. As women, we tend to nurture those around us, often neglecting our own needs. Now is the time to be selfish, be strong, and be smart. I wholeheartedly wish you courage and strength to face breast cancer (or any of life's adversities). To quote Robert Frost, "The best way out is always through."

PART II

. . . .

Complementary Cancer Treatment

. . . .

14.

NUTRITIONAL THERAPY

. . . .

A diagnosis of breast cancer prompts many women to reevaluate their dietary practices as they wonder what caused this cancer to occur and what lifestyle changes they should make to ensure recovery or prevent recurrence. While proper nutrition can help boost your immune system and maintain health both during and after treatment, it is only one of several lifestyle factors you should consider. Exercise and stress management can work in conjunction with your diet to increase your overall health and well-being. See chapter 15 for suggestions on low-impact movement therapies such as yoga and qigong and mind/body therapies such as meditation and breathwork.

For breast cancer treatment, the elements of nutritional therapy can range from adjustments in caloric intake and the kinds of foods in your diet to vitamin and mineral supplementation. For example, people with breast cancer frequently require a diet high in calories and protein to prevent weight loss and muscle wasting during treatment. For those attempting to avoid recurrence, fruits, vegetables, and whole grains are known to contain phytochemicals with antioxidant, antiestrogen, and chemopreventive properties that may prevent cancer. Also, high doses of vitamin C are often used to aid in breast cancer treatment and to assist the healing of scar tissue that often results from surgery.

However, as with any complementary therapy, you must consult with your physician before implementing any nutritional therapy. Many vitamins and supplements may be contraindicated for some cancer medications and could interfere with treatment. For example, taking vitamin C in tablet form during chemotherapy with Adriamycin will prevent the chemotherapy from working properly. This chapter will outline some of the most promising nutritional therapies available to breast cancer patients, which you may want to explore further with your physician.

Recommended Reading
Beating Cancer With Nutrition, by Patrick Quillen and Noreen Quillen (Bookworld Services, 2001).

VITAMINS AND MINERALS

Vitamins and minerals, necessary for the continued life and health of any organism, are an important part of a balanced diet. In various shapes, forms, and preparations, vitamin and mineral supplements have been used for thousands of years and by different cultures and civilizations in the fight against diseases, cancers, and the promotion of vitality and long life. Modern medicine has begun to recognize the need to evaluate vitamins and minerals in terms of their potential value and benefit to all types of patients.

A strong note of caution regarding the use of vitamin and mineral supplements, and nutritional supplements in general: It is imperative that you discuss any questions or considerations about supplements with your doctor before you take any over-the-counter substances. Many of the common supplements have important and possibly deadly interactions with some medications, and may affect you directly. Also, remember that the Food and Drug Administration does not supervise the dietary supplement market in the United States, and the quality and contents of these substances varies widely among manufacturers. Many supplements are manufactured outside of the United States, where no quality control supervision exists. Dosage recommendations are not provided here, because you should discuss with your doctor your potential usage on an individual basis.

Recommended Reading

Fight Cancer with Vitamins and Supplements: A Guide to Prevention and Treatment, by Kedar N. Prasad, Ph.D., and Frank L. Meyskens, Jr. (Inner Traditions International, 2001).

Antioxidants Against Cancer, by Ralph W. Moss (Equinox Press, 2000).

Vitamin A and Beta-Carotene

Vitamin A is essential for maintaining the proper functions of many body systems, including the immune system, the skin, and the eyes, and it helps protect the body from cardiovascular disease and cancer. Vitamin A is stored in the liver, and extremely large doses can be toxic. A compound of vitamin A, beta-carotene, is easily converted into vitamin A in the body as needed and has no potential toxic effects.

Dietary sources of vitamin A are only found in animal products such as fish liver oil of cod, halibut, salmon, and shark; eggs; and dairy products. Beta-carotene is found in green and yellow-orange fruits and vegetables such as apricots, cantaloupe, carrots, parsley, and spinach. However, heat can eliminate the effectiveness of both vitamin A and beta-carotene, and supplementation is often recommended.

Benefits

Many studies have shown that vitamin A can help reduce the risk of many cancers, including breast cancer. Vitamin A is also useful in the treatment of existing breast cancer (and other cancers) by slowing metastasis and enhancing the effectiveness of chemotherapy.

Vitamin C (Ascorbic Acid)

Vitamin C is essential for healthy teeth, gums, and bones, and is required for the synthesis of collagen, the intercellular "cement" that holds tissues together. It is also one of the major antioxidant nutrients, and it prevents the conversion of nitrates (for example, from tobacco smoke, smog, bacon, lunch meats, and some vegetables) into cancer-causing substances. Dr. Linus Pauling, the foremost authority on vitamin C, claimed that proper vitamin C intake can decrease the risk of getting certain cancers by 75 percent. The primary sources of vitamin C are broccoli, Brussels sprouts, cabbage, cauliflower, kale, lemon pulp, melons, okra, orange pulp, tangerines, and turnip greens.

Benefits

Vitamin C has many uses in the treatment of side effects associated with cancer and cancer treatment: it can help heal wounds and scar tissue, and it builds resistance to infection (common among chemotherapy patients), strengthens the immune system against the common cold, and gives strength to blood vessels. Vitamin C has shown particular effectiveness in the treatment of malignant cancers, specifically bladder cancer, breast cancer, and cancer of the colon.

Vitamin D

Vitamin D, a fat-soluble vitamin, is used in the absorption of calcium. Vitamin D is formed in the skin of animals and humans by the action of shortwave ultraviolet light, the so-called fast-tanning sun rays.

Benefits

Evidence of vitamin D's protective effect against cancer is compelling. Tumor cells are young, immortal cells that never mature or die off. Vitamin D derivatives have been shown to promote normal cell growth and maturation, prompting researchers to attempt to engineer forms of vitamin D for anticancer therapy.

Vitamin E

Vitamin E is found in foods such as vegetable oils and shortening, meat, eggs, milk, and leafy vegetables, and it can be taken in capsule or liquid form. It is used in the body by almost all tissues and is stored primarily in fat and muscle tissue. Vitamin E has been proven to prolong the life of cells and to help maintain organ function. Do not take more vitamin E than is prescribed for you or than is directed on the package as too much can be dangerous.

Benefits

Vitamin E is a powerful antioxidant and effectively protects the heart, boosts immunity, heals wounds, and preserves brain tissue. Most important for cancer patients, however, is that vitamin E is also an anticarcinogen. Studies have shown vitamin E to play not only a role in cancer prevention but also in treatment, as it may reduce the size of tumors and protect normal cells during aggressive treatment.

Vitamin K

Vitamin K is a fat-soluble vitamin that plays an important role in blood clotting. Vitamin K supplementation is often unnecessary, since it is synthesized in the body and is easily obtained from a regular diet that includes broccoli, green cabbage, liver, spinach, and tomatoes.

Benefits

Vitamin K can help improve the survival of cancer patients as it has been shown to reduce the metastasis of cancer and protect against tumor growth, especially when used in conjunction with radiation therapy.

Cesium and Rubidium

Cesium and rubidium are colloidal ionic minerals, taken orally as dietary supplements.

Benefits

Cesium and rubidium act as catalysts for other nutrients, vitamins, hormones, and neurological functions. When taken, it is believed they alkalinize cancer cells (by neutralizing their acid nature, thereby increasing pH levels). Cancer cells cannot survive in the higher pH ranges and die off.

Molybdenum

Molybdenum is a silver-gray metal. Its name is derived from the Greek word "molybdaena," meaning "lead." Taken orally as a dietary supplement, it is an antioxidant.

Benefits

Antioxidants have been shown to prevent cancer, and are generally devoid of the major toxic side effects of many current anticancer drugs.

Selenium

Selenium is a potent antioxidant that protects the body from damage due to oxidation by free radicals. It is a trace element, or micronutrient, since the amount needed for human health is measured in micrograms (millionths of a gram). In excess, selenium can be toxic. Aside from dietary supplements, the following foods are excellent sources of selenium: brazil nuts, wheat germ, molasses, sunflower seeds, whole-wheat bread, and dairy foods.

Benefits

Selenium works with vitamin E and other antioxidants to protect cells from damage, synthesize antibodies and coenzyme Q10, and transport ions across cell membranes.

SUPPLEMENTS

Cartilage (Bovine and Shark)

Cartilage, derived from shark and bovine (cow) sources, is a type of connective tissue comprised of mucopolysaccharides, protein substances, calcium, sulfur, and collagen. Cartilage is a food supplement that is taken orally in powder or tablet form. Bovine cartilage is typically recommended at 3 grams 3 times per day. Shark cartilage is typically taken in much higher amounts (i.e., 60 to 100 grams per day orally or by enema). These amounts are based on animal and anecdotal evidence, and their safety and efficacy have not been confirmed by controlled clinical trials. Not only is toxicity information on this amount of shark cartilage lacking, but also the amount of calcium to be found in this amount of shark cartilage exceeds the 2 to 2.5 grams per day that is commonly considered to be the upper limit of safe intake. Cartilage itself has no known toxicity. However, it has been known to cause nausea and indigestion in some patients.

Benefits

Cartilage has been investigated for its potential role in regulating immune functions and stopping the growth of tumors. The role of shark cartilage in inhibiting the growth of new blood vessels (angiogenesis) is theorized to be beneficial in halting the growth and spread of cancer. In the United States, there have been a few clinical trials with high doses of IV shark cartilage. So far, the results have been inconclusive.

Coenzyme Q10

Coenzyme Q10 (CoQ10) is one in a series of ubiquinones—naturally occurring compounds produced in nearly every cell of the body and found in almost all cells, but levels decrease as we age. It's also found in most foods, though in tiny amounts. It helps convert food into energy at a very basic, cellular level, and it is an antioxidant. Coenzyme Q10 is taken orally.

Supplementation should be continued long term because it may require 8 weeks or longer to notice results.

Benefits
Researchers are investigating the possible antioxidant benefits of coenzyme Q10 in helping to fight breast cancer and other diseases linked to free-radical damage. A few small studies suggest that coenzyme Q10 may prolong survival in those with breast or prostate cancer, though results remain inconclusive. It's also used as a general energy enhancer and antiaging supplement. Because levels of the compound diminish with age (and with certain diseases), some doctors recommend daily supplementation beginning around age 40.

Recommended Reading
The Miracle Nutrient: Coenzyme Q10, by Emile G. Bliznakov, M.D., and Gerry Hunt (Bantam Books, 1987).

Algae
Algae are photosynthetic organisms that occur in most habitats, ranging from marine and fresh water to desert sands, and from hot boiling springs to snow and ice. They vary from small, single-celled forms to complex multicellular forms. Ocean/sea algae are the richest natural source of minerals, trace minerals, and rare earth elements. They are usually sold dry in health food stores. Algae are ingested orally. Capsules are available, but many people cook delicious dishes incorporating algae.

Benefits
Algae are a rich source of iodine, selenium, organic geranium, calcium, iron, silicon, copper, and zinc, many of which are effective anticancer nutrients.

Recommended Reading
Earth Food Spirulina: How This Remarkable Blue-Green Algae Can Transform Your Health and Our Planet, by Robert Henrikson (Ronore Enterprises, 1997).

Canthaxanthin
Canthaxanthin is a well-studied carotenoid (a family of natural pigments found in plants and animals) widely distributed throughout nature.

Canthaxanthin comes from a type of edible mushroom and from the feathers of the flamingo. It is used as a food-coloring agent, and it also is sold as a tanning pill. Canthaxanthin makes your stool red and leaves an orange tinge on the palms of your hands and the soles of your feet. Hepatitis and allergic skin reactions may result from its use. It has also been reported to occasionally cause damage to the eye.

Benefits

Supporters argue that canthaxanthin may boost your immune system by neutralizing free radicals, which are believed to lead to cancer. Supporters of canthaxanthin claim that it is helpful with breast cancer.

Indoles

Indoles are a family of chemicals from the cruciferous vegetables that are named for the cross shape of their four-petal flowers. They can be consumed in broccoli, Brussels sprouts, cabbage, cauliflower, kale, kohlrabi, mustard greens, rutabagas, and turnips.

Benefits

Indoles are widely touted for their anticancer properties, and research suggests that they stimulate enzymes that make estrogen less effective in promoting tumor growth.

Linseed Oil (Flaxseed Oil)

Linseed oil is amber-colored fatty oil extracted from the cotyledons and inner coats of the linseed. Linseed oil has long been used as a drying oil in paints and varnish and in making linoleum, oilcloth, and certain inks.

Benefits

Linseed oil can stop the development of many forms of cancer and relieve many of the side effects associated with cancer and its treatment. It has been proven to help prevent hair loss and encourage hair growth (after a year of usage), increase energy and stamina, help treat depression, and shorten the recovery time of fatigued muscles.

Recommended Reading

Flaxseed (Linseed) Oil and the Power of Omega-3, by James R. Johnston (Keats, 1989).

Mushrooms

There are several varieties of edible mushrooms, including portobello, cremini, and button. Most mushroom products sold as supplements are combinations of 3 to 10 medicinal mushrooms, many originating in China. In Japan and China, certain mushrooms have even been approved as cancer-fighting drugs.

Benefits

A study presented at the Twenty-second Annual San Antonio Breast Cancer Symposium suggests that certain foods, such as mushrooms, contain naturally occurring chemicals that inhibit an enzyme known as aromatase. Aromatase is a key enzyme in the body involved in estrogen synthesis, and research suggests that inhibition of this enzyme can slow breast cancer growth. Some mushroom extracts, particularly shiitake, may reduce the side effects of chemotherapy and radiation therapy.

Recommended Reading

Medicinal Benefits of Mushrooms: Healing for More Than Twenty Centuries— Their Effects on Cancer, Diabetes, Heart Disease and More, by William H. R. Lee, Ph.D. (Keats, 1997).

SOY

• • • • • •

Although soy foods are widely recognized for their nutritional qualities, interest in soy has risen recently because scientists have discovered that a component in it called "isoflavanes" appears to reduce the risk of breast cancer and to block estrogen from cancer cells. Soy is also often recommended to reduce the occurrence and severity of hot flashes that are often a side effect of hormonal therapy.

The more popular soy foods, such as tofu, meat alternatives, soy sauce, soy flour, and soybean oil, can be found in supermarkets. The greatest variety of soy foods can be found in natural and health foods stores and Asian markets. Several products, such as textured soy flour, textured soy protein concentrates, soy nuts, and soy nut butter, can be obtained through mail-order catalogs.

15.

COMPLEMENTARY &
ALTERNATIVE MEDICINE

. . . .

Complementary medicine covers a wide range of approaches, including various philosophies of healing and many types of therapies. Some therapies are termed "holistic," meaning that good health involves the well-being of all aspects of a person: physical, mental, spiritual, and emotional. Many of these therapies are termed "preventative," meaning the complementary care provider educates and provides the tools to keep health problems from arising. Complementary care works best when you, your physician, and the complementary care practitioner act together to help get you well and stay well.

An increasing number of breast cancer patients are turning to complementary therapies as part of their overall cancer treatment plan. An "alternative" therapy is a treatment that is used in place of traditional medicine. A "complementary" therapy (also called integrative medicine, or CAM) is a treatment that is used as a supplement to traditional medicine. When properly combined with standard cancer treatments, some complementary therapies can enhance wellness and quality of life. This chapter will outline some of the most effective, promising, and commonly used CAM therapies for breast cancer patients.

Before selecting a complementary or alternative therapy, it is essential to consider:

- The safety and effectiveness of the therapy or treatment.
- The expertise and qualifications of the health care practitioner.
- The quality of the service delivery.

It is important for patients to realize that not all alternative or complementary medicines are safe. Patients who are considering nontraditional medicines should thoroughly investigate the therapy and consult with their physicians or alternative medicine practitioners to make sure the therapy is safe and will not interact with other medicines they may be taking. Some therapies may interact negatively with your prescribed treatment plan.

Note: No form of integrative medicine (CAM) treatment should be utilized without full disclosure/collaboration with your physician/integrative medicine team. All integrative medicine providers should be licensed or certified where license/certification exists, which will often depend on the state or country in which you reside. Safety and efficacy of individual integrative therapies should always be discussed with your integrative medicine provider and physician prior to initiating treatment.

A QUICK COMPARISON OF EASTERN AND WESTERN MEDICINE VIEWPOINTS

The fundamental philosophies behind Eastern and Western medicine are quite different. In Western medical practice and theory, reliability and power are essential, and the best drug is considered to be the one that has the most immediate effects. In modern Western science, every single cell of a body is thought to be a function of the human body. So, a good medicine is required to have quick effects on the affected parts of the body, and is prescribed for treatment even if it contains slight toxicity.

Contrastingly, in Eastern health systems, medications with fewer side effects are preferred. To improve and strengthen the body, spontaneous cure and long-term inner balance are considered more important than fast, short-lived effects. The main idea behind Eastern medical science is that the main role of any remedy is to help improve the total body condition.

Both Western and Eastern medications can help us recover from illness and maintain best health conditions. What is important for us is not to necessarily choose one of the two but to acquaint ourselves with the merits and demerits of both, and to use them effectively.

HOW TO CHOOSE A PRACTITIONER

In the United States, CAM practitioners typically specialize in a particular component of alternative medicine such as acupuncture, herbal therapy, or massage, rather than an entire discipline. The regulation of practitioners varies from state to state. Acupuncturists are licensed in many states, and Doctors of Oriental Medicine (O.M.D.) are licensed in some states to prescribe herbal remedies as well as acupuncture treatments. Many biomedically trained doctors, naturopaths, osteopaths, and chiropractors have studied acupuncture and other CAM therapies and incorporated them into their practices.

Mastering the full range of CAM is a complex process that requires many years of study and practice. However, medical personnel with less training may still be able to perform acupuncture and herbal medicine safely by working according to protocols designed by alternative medicine practitioners. As you would with any health care provider, check into your CAM practitioner's training and background.

Things to consider
- If you have a chronic condition or a new acute problem that is seriously disabling you, get a diagnostic evaluation from a conventional primary care physician before consulting a CAM practitioner.
- Plan on coordinating your care between your biomedical doctor and your CAM practitioner. If they won't work together, find ones that will.
- As with any health care practitioner, if the condition is not improving in a reasonable amount of time, obtain a second opinion. There are increasing numbers of practitioners familiar with both Western medicine and CAM, should you need a reevaluation.

AROMATHERAPY

Aromatherapy is the art and science of utilizing naturally extracted aromatic essences from plants to balance, harmonize, and promote the health of body, mind, and spirit. It is a natural, noninvasive treatment system designed to affect the whole person, not just the symptom or disease, and to assist the body's natural ability to balance, regulate, heal, and maintain itself by the correct use of essential oils. Essential oils are pure, concentrated plant extracts obtained specifically for their fragrance and therapeutic value. The chemical composition of these oils is exceedingly complex—they often involve tens or hundreds of constituent parts. Essential oils are readily available from many health food and aromatherapy stores, via mail order, and via companies that have websites. Although they are readily available, the quality of essential oils from one vendor to another can vary drastically, whether you buy them locally or not.

What to Expect

Pure essential oils are blended for harmonious, combined effect and fragrance. Skillful blending balances the therapeutic effect and aromatic quality of individual essential oils. The scent of essential oils is conveyed by the olfactory nerve to areas of the brain that can influence emotions and hormonal response. When used in a bath or massage, the oils are absorbed through the skin and carried by body fluids to the main body systems such as the nervous and muscular systems for a healing effect. It is most beneficial to go to an aromatherapy practitioner who is skilled in massage and well versed in essential oils. However, aromatherapy can be practiced at home safely and effectively.

How to use essential oils:

- Place a few drops of essential oil into a bowl of steaming water. Breathe the steam for 15 to 30 minutes. This is great for clearing sinuses and providing head cold relief.
- Place a drop or two on your wrist. Breathe it while you work. When you have had enough, wash it off. (This is like wearing perfume.)
- Place a few drops on a cloth. Use this cloth as a scarf or place it on your pillowcase. Move cloth away when you have had enough. (Great to use while sleeping.)
- Use during massage. This can have amazing effects. Beware that changes can happen extremely fast when doing this, so dilution is recommended.

Benefits

There are two primary ways to benefit from aromatherapy: by breathing the aromatic vapors using an aroma diffuser or air freshener, or by absorbing diluted oils through the skin in a bath or massage. Emotion-based benefits include relief of depression, grief, hysteria, anxiety, fear, sadness, and insomnia. Medicinal benefits include relief of fatigue, motion sickness, burns, and muscular aches, and enhanced wound healing.

Aromatherapy is helpful in easing the physical and emotional effects of breast cancer treatments.

- *Frankincense:* for calming emotions.
- *Lavender:* for relaxation.
- *Peppermint:* for quick energy.
- *Sandalwood:* for relaxation, digestive troubles (especially due to tension), dry skin (especially after radiation).
- *Tea tree:* strong disinfectant, antibacterial, and antifungal.

Recommended Reading

The Complete Book of Essential Oils and Aromatherapy, by Valerie Ann Worwood (New World Library, 1991).

AYURVEDA

Ayurveda is an ancient Indian medical practice that encompasses a range of treatments, including medicinal herbs, changes in diet, meditation, massage, and yoga, to maintain or restore health. The word *Ayurveda* is Sanskrit and means "science (or knowledge) of life." It recognizes the unique differences of all individuals and therefore recommends different regimens for different types of people. Although two people may appear to have the same outward symptoms, their energetic constitutions may be very different and therefore call for very different remedies.

According to Ayurveda, every person contains some of the universe's five basic elements: earth, air, fire, water, and ether (or space). The combination of these elements in each individual breaks down into three metabolic body types, or *doshas.* The doshas are known as *vata, pitta,* and *kapha.* Vata consists of ether and air and is associated with lightness and movement. Pitta is made of fire and is associated with transformative metabolic processes—the digestion of food to produce energy, for example. Kapha consists of earth and water and is associated with structure and stability.

What to Expect

Once the causes of an illness are identified, measures can be taken by an individual, under the guidance of an Ayurvedic practitioner, to restore balance and to remove toxicity. A first visit to an Ayurvedic practitioner may last 45 to 90 minutes. The practitioner will ask a series of questions to determine your doshic profile. The practitioner will listen to your heart and lungs and pay special attention to your pulses and tongue. After identifying your doshic type and any imbalances, the physician may prescribe a combination of Ayurvedic treatments, including herbal remedies, lifestyle and dietary modifications (vegetarianism is not required), meditation and yoga postures, breathing exercises, and cleansing measures such as nasal douching or enemas.

Benefits

Ayurveda eliminates disease from the root; there are few, if any, side effects (which are common with modern drugs); it offers long-term cure with all-natural herbal remedies (no toxic chemicals or animal products); and therapy is effective and inexpensive.

Recommended Reading

Ayurveda for Women, by Dr. Robert E. Svoboda (Inner Traditions International, 2000).

BODYWORK

Bodywork is the treatment of the human body/mind/spirit—including the electromagnetic or energetic field, which surrounds, infuses, and brings that body to life—by pressure and/or manipulation. Bodywork is based on techniques and treatment strategies to primarily affect and balance the energetic system for the purpose of treating the human body, emotions, mind, energy field, and spirit, or for the promotion, maintenance, and restoration of health.

Benefits
- Relaxation and stress management.
- Drug-free pain relief.
- Facilitation of healing.
- Promotion of circulation of blood, lymph, and *chi* (vital energy).
- Improved flexibility, mobility, and posture.
- Increased focus, awareness, performance, creativity, vitality, and self-esteem.
- Complementary to other forms of care such as chiropractic, acupuncture, psychotherapy, dentistry, and Western medical treatments with or without medication.
- Some massage therapy has been shown to decrease fatigue during chemotherapy.

Recommended Reading

The Encyclopedia of Bodywork: From Acupressure to Zone Therapy, by Elaine Stillerman (Facts on File, 1996).

Massage

Massage is the manipulation of the soft tissues of the body with the hands for therapeutic, healing, relaxing, and pleasurable effects. Massages and other touch therapies are great for releasing accumulated stress and removing blocks from the system—both physical as well as psychological.

What to Expect

Your session will begin with your therapist asking you about your reasons for getting a massage, your current physical condition, your brief medical history, your lifestyle and stress level, and any areas of pain you may have. You'll be asked to undress in private, down to your underwear or to whatever amount of clothing you feel comfortable wearing. You may also choose to stay fully clothed. Then, lying down on a comfortably padded massage table, you'll drape yourself with a sheet and blanket. Only the part of the body being worked on is uncovered, and your modesty is respected.

You can expect a peaceful and comfortable environment for the massage. For the period of time agreed on, typically 30 to 60 minutes, all of your muscles will be kneaded in a full-body massage—or only in specific areas, in the case of a session oriented to localized injury, pain or tightness, or sports readiness. A well-trained massage therapist should not only apply a variety of techniques to address your particular needs but also exude a calm, respectful, nonjudgmental demeanor to allow a sense of trust to develop between client and therapist. Make sure you tell the practitioner about any injuries or medical problems you currently have.

Physical Benefits
- Helps relieve muscle tension and stiffness.
- Increases white blood cells and natural killer cell activity, suggesting a benefit to the immune system.
- Helps relieve stress and aids relaxation.
- Reduces pain and swelling; reduces formation of excessive scar tissue.
- Promotes deeper and easier breathing.
- Reduces heart rate, lowers blood pressure.
- Improves circulation of blood and movement of lymph fluids.
- Postoperative rehabilitation.

Mental Benefits
- Promotes a relaxed state of mental alertness.
- Helps relieve mental stress.
- Satisfies needs for caring, nurturing touch.
- Fosters a feeling of well-being.
- Reduces levels of anxiety.
- Creates body awareness.

Recommended Reading
Medicine Hands: Massage Therapy for People with Cancer, by Gayle MacDonald (Findhorn Press, 1999).

Acupressure
Acupressure is the no-needle next of kin of the more popular Chinese therapy of acupuncture (see "Traditional Chinese Medicine" on page 168). In acupressure, the emphasis is on curing through proper pressure on concerned nerve points in the human body. An acupressurist works with the same points used in acupuncture to release blocked energy, but stimulates these healing sites with finger pressure, rather than by inserting fine needles.

What to Expect

You will lie fully clothed on a soft massage table while the practitioner presses gently on points on various parts of your body. By using deep but gentle finger pressure on specific points, the blocked energy is released, allowing your body/mind to relax. As your body/mind relaxes, you have an opportunity to explore thought patterns, memories, and belief systems. Through mindful exploration, the way you experience your universe can change, allowing you an opportunity to manifest your purpose in life with less discomfort and stress and with a greater sense of well-being.

The session is noninvasive and gentle. An average session lasts for about an hour. Most clients normally require a number of sessions to complete a treatment.

Benefits

Using the power and sensitivity of the hand, acupressure is effective in the relief of stress-related ailments, in self-treatment, and in preventive health care. Acupressure can also be combined with massage to release tension, reduce pain, increase blood circulation, and develop vibrant health. All of these benefits can be particularly useful to a woman with breast cancer.

Recommended Reading

Living Pain Free with Acupressure, by Dr. Devi S. Nambudripad (Delta, 1997).

Alexander Technique

The Alexander Technique works to change habits in the way you perform everyday activities. It is a simple and practical method for improving ease and freedom of movement, balance, support, and coordination. The technique teaches the use of the appropriate amount of effort for a particular activity, giving you more energy for all your activities. It is not a series of treatments or exercises but rather a reeducation of the mind and body.

What to Expect

For a start, you don't remove your clothes and no special clothing is required. Alexander lessons are not painful—there is nothing physically aggressive about the work. During the lesson, your teacher will observe your posture and movement patterns as you perform simple movements such as walking, standing, or sitting. She will also supplement the visual informa- tion by using her hands, gently placing them on your neck, shoulders, and back, to get more refined information about your patterns of breathing and moving. The teacher's hands will gently guide your body to encourage a release of restrictive muscular tension.

A lesson usually lasts between 30 and 45 minutes. It will probably take a few lessons for you and your teacher to get an idea of how quickly you will make progress. As with learning other new skills, a lot depends on how far you want to take it. The majority of students go for a few months, taking between 20 and 40 lessons during that period, and then perhaps return for refresher lessons or groups of lessons from time to time.

Benefits

The Alexander Technique works by finding different ways of moving that are easier and more efficient, therefore decreasing wear and tear on body structures and internal organs. It also helps detect and let go of excessive tension that has been held unconsciously in the body. The benefits of this technique are that it significantly decreases physical and mental stress and improves breathing. This can often be particularly helpful for breast cancer patients after reconstructive surgery, along with Feldenkrais and Pilates.

Recommended Reading

The Alexander Technique Manual: A Step-by-Step Guide to Improve Breathing, Posture, and Well-Being, by Richard Brennan (Charles Tuttle, 1996).

Feldenkrais

The Feldenkrais method is a mind/body integration technique that uses movement to enhance the communication between the brain and the body. With an increased awareness and correction of physical habits that strain joints and muscles, improved physical and mental performance is achieved, as well as a more positive self-image and better overall health.

What to Expect

Moshe Feldenkrais developed over 1,000 different movements or exercises that are taught in one of two approaches. Private one-on-one sessions focus on hands-on touch and guided movement that is called Functional Integration. Group lessons are called Awareness Through Movement. In both types of sessions, pupils (not patients) are guided by teachers through a series of slow, gentle sequences of movements designed to replace old, negative habits with new, positive ones. At no time is any attempt made to alter the structure of the body. Instead, a series of slow, nonaerobic, and often quirky and subtle movements are repeated over and over, concentrating on only one body segment or joint at a time.

Benefits

The body is then taught how to function with greater ease, fluidity, and motion, resulting in better health and an improved self-image. Healthy students generally experience improved posture and relief of muscular tension following a session. They also report better flexibility and coordination. This method is also used to alleviate chronic pain often associated with breast cancer, to reduce stress and tension, and to improve balance and coordination.

Recommended Reading

Awareness Heals: The Feldenkrais Method for Dynamic Health, by Steven Shafarman (Perseus Press, 1997).

Reflexology

Reflexology is a science based on the premise that there are zones and reflex areas in the feet and hands that correspond to all glands, organs, parts, and systems of the body. The physical act of applying pressure using thumb, finger, and hand techniques to these areas results in the reduction of stress, which promotes physiological changes in the body.

What to Expect

Reflexology is a hands-on practice. There are zones throughout the body that are most accessible within the feet and hands. Client safety as well as efficacy of application can best be served by the use of the practitioner's hands, fingers, and thumbs. The use of oils, lotions, and creams before or during the application of reflexology is strongly discouraged, as such use only serves to blur the lines between reflexology and massage as well as to interfere with sensory feedback.

Benefits

Not only does reflexology reduce nervous tension and thereby induce a deep state of relaxation, but it also increases vitality by releasing energy trapped in tense parts of the body. Reflexology treatment improves the circulation of the blood, and this facilitates the better transport of both nutrients around the body and waste products to the organs of elimination. Many health problems have been successfully treated by reflexology, including stress, fatigue, anxiety (common symptoms and side effects of breast cancer), insomnia, constipation, and back and shoulder pain.

Recommended Reading
Reflexology for Every Body, by Joan Cosway-Hayes (Footloose Press, 1999).

Reiki

Reiki is a Japanese energy healing system based on the belief that thoughts have the power to direct energy—the underlying dynamo shaping the world. Reiki is made up of two words—"rei" and "ki." "Rei" can be interpreted as a higher form of intelligence, while "ki" is yet another spelling of *chi* or qi—life force. Often described as a form of Shinto-Buddhist qigong, Reiki was rediscovered by Dr. Mikao Usui in the early twentieth century.

Dr. Usui adopted five admonitions to live by that, if applied with Reiki, would heal the body, bring peace of mind, and bring happiness in life. These admonitions are taught as the *Reiki Principles:*

1. Don't get angry today.
2. Don't be grievous.
3. Express your thanks.
4. Be diligent in your business.
5. Be kind to others.

What to Expect

Reiki is a multidimensional energy healing system that works by raising the vibrations of the being or object to be healed closer to those of the practitioner. Reiki is transferred to students by Reiki Masters through a series of attunements. During an attunement process, the Master selects a series of symbols that represent important points located along a person's energy field and guides them through higher vibrations of energy. This attunement process enables recipients to access the healing energy on their own, which can heal the cause of a problem at whatever level it may exist—body, mind, or spirit.

Benefits
Reiki is of great benefit for:

- Supporting conventional medicine and minimizing the side effects of drugs.
- Support during times of crises, depression, illness, death, and bereavement.
- Stimulating the natural healing of acute and chronic ailments.
- Speeding recovery after surgery and injury.
- Managing stress and tension.
- Releasing blocked energies and cleansing toxins.
- Perception of inner clarity, wisdom, intuition, awareness, and enlightenment.
- Promoting harmony within relationships.

Recommended Reading
The Original Reiki Handbook, by Mikao Usui and Frank Arjava Petter (Lotus Press, 1999).

BOWEN THERAPY

Bowen therapy is a simple holistic therapy that balances and integrates the body's systems. Bowen Therapy is not massage, chiropractic, or acupressure, but rather a system of stimulating body reflexes. Simple yet precise movements are executed across muscles, nerves, and connective tissue at a series of key points on the body; it stimulates energy flow that releases tension, strains, and blockages, empowering the body's own resources to naturally rebalance and heal itself. The relief is profound and lasting, affecting muscular, digestive, respiratory, glandular, and energetic systems. Tom Bowen developed this therapy in Australia between the mid-1950s and early 1980s. There are currently 60 teachers offering seminars around the globe.

What to Expect

A Bowen session consists of a series of gentle movements of hands on skin (or through light clothing), with the client usually lying on a bed or treatment couch. Each session lasts approximately 30 to 45 minutes. In many cases, longstanding pain can be relieved in 2 to 3 sessions, although further treatments may be required in some situations There is no manipulation or adjustment of hard tissue; the treatment is very gentle, relaxing, and safe for all ages.

Benefits

The Bowen technique encourages a gentle response, which empowers the body's own resources to heal itself. The results are usually a deep sense of overall relaxation, allowing the body to recharge and balance itself.

Recommended Reading

The Bowen Technique, by Julian Baker (Human Kinetics, 2002).

Additional resources:

Bowen Research and Training Institute
Connell Square
38541 U.S. Highway 19 North
Palm Harbor, FL 34684
www.bowen.org/bowen/
(727) 937-9077

In Europe:

European College of Bowen Therapy
38 Portway, Frome, Somerset
England BA11 1QU
www.thebowentechnique.com
44 (0)1373 461873

COLOR THERAPY

Color therapy is based on the fact that physiologic functions respond to specific colors. Therapists believe that color has an effect on each of us.

Therapists use this approach to restore cells to an even level of balance and to stimulate the healing processes. Because colors can have both a positive and negative effect, specific colors and accurate amounts of color are critical in healing.

What to Expect

Color therapy can be practiced with either colored light or color pigments such as paints or swatches.

Here is a guide to specific colors and their effects.

- *Black:* self-confidence, power, strength.
- *Blue:* calming, lowers blood pressure, decreases respiration.
- *Green:* soothing, relaxing mentally as well as physically, helps those suffering from depression, anxiety, nervousness.
- *Violet:* suppresses appetite, provides a peaceful environment, good for migraines.
- *Pink:* used in diet therapy as an appetite suppressant, relaxes muscles, relieves tension, soothing.
- *Yellow:* energizes, relieves depression, improves memory, and stimulates appetite.
- *Orange:* energizes, stimulates appetite and digestive system.
- *Red:* stimulates brain wave activity, increases heart rate, respirations, and blood pressure, excites sexual glands.

Benefits

Exposing the body to colored light is also believed to aid in healing. Specifially, green light is believed to help heart problems and cancer.

Recommended Reading

Color Therapy: Healing with Color, by Reuben Amber (Aurora Press, 1983).

ELECTROMAGNETISM

Electromagnetism describes the relationship between electricity and magnetism and works on the principle that an electric current through a wire generates a magnetic field. In a wire, the magnetic field forms around the wire. If the wire is wrapped around a metal object, it can often magnetize that object, making an electromagnet. Electromagnets are used in many therapies that can be useful in the treatment of cancer, including electric therapy, heat therapy, and magnetic therapy.

Electric Therapy

Electrotherapy, also known as electrochemical tumor therapy, Galvanotherapy, and electrocancer treatment (ECT), was developed in Europe by the Swedish professor Björn Nordenström and the Austrian doctor Rudolf Pekar. The therapy employs galvanic electrical stimulation to treat tumors and skin cancers; ECT is used most often as an adjunct with other therapies.

What to Expect

Using local anesthesia, the physician inserts a positively charged platinum, gold, or silver needle into the tumor and places negatively charged needles around the tumor. Voltages of 6 to 15 volts are used, depending on tumor size. To enhance the cancer cell–killing power of ECT, small amounts of chemotherapy agents can be applied to the skin and driven into the tumor by a kind of sweating effect of the electric current.

Benefits

This therapy depolarizes cancer cell membranes and causes tumors to be gently destroyed. The process also appears to generate heat shock proteins around the cancer cells, inducing cell-specific immunity.

Heat Therapy

Heat therapy increases the temperature in a selected area of the body. For basic aches and pains, first apply heat to the affected area. Moist heat from a warm shower or hydrocollator can reduce stiffness and relax muscles. After heat has been applied, firmly rub and massage the affected area; this will also relieve tension.

Benefits

Heat enhances blood circulation and increases mobility.

Magnetic Therapy

Magnetic therapy is the application of magnetic fields on parts of the body to speed healing, decrease relative pain and inflammation, and improve bodily functions. It simulates the earth's magnetic field and places your body in an optimum environment to heal itself.

What to Expect
Magnets, or low-voltage charges, are placed around the body to "recharge" the energy fields. Additionally, magnetics and low voltage are used to oxygenate the body's tissues. This particular therapy is often used in conjunction with oxygen therapies as well as augmenting others.

Benefits
Magnetic therapy is often used to treat backaches, burns, chronic fatigue syndrome, insomnia, migraines, and poor circulation, among other ailments. For breast cancer patients, magnetic therapy has proven effective in reducing pain, promoting sleep, and reducing stress. What makes magnets so attractive are their effectiveness, ease of use, low cost, and durability, and the absence of side effects.

Recommended Reading
Magnet Therapy: The Pain Cure Alternative, by Ron Lawrence, Judith Plowden, and Paul J. Rosch (Prima, 1998).

ESSIAC

Essiac (es-ee-ack) is an herbal tea remedy attributed to the Canadian nurse Rene M. Caisse, who claimed the source of her recipe was an old Indian medicine man. Rene treated cancer patients with her Essiac remedy for 50 years. Her *Rene M. Caisse Cancer Clinic* functioned from 1935 until 1941. Rene Caisse named her herbal remedy "Essiac" after the backward spelling of her last name.

What to Expect
Find a commercial product made by an ethical marketer or get into making your own essiac tea if you have the time and want to save a lot of money. Avoid essiac capsules and dunkable tea bags because they are usually made with raw herbs and not traditional brewing. Essiac tinctures and extracts are made by steeping the raw herbs in alcohol or nonsoluble glycerin

(but their convenience makes them popular). These are the four herbs that you use to make essiac tea:

- Burdock root (Arctium lappa)
- Sheep sorrel (Rumex acetosella)
- Turkey rhubarb root (Rheum palmatum)
- Slippery elm bark (Ulmus fulva)

Benefits

Proponents of Essiac claim that it strengthens the immune system, improves appetite, relieves pain, and improves overall quality of life. They also claim that it shrinks tumors and prolongs the lives of people with cancer. There is no scientific evidence that proves that Rene Caisse's formula cures, alleviates, or prevents any disease or condition. There are no known interactions between Essiac and medications or other herbs. However, most interactions between herbs and medications have not been studied. Tell your doctor if you are using herbal supplements.

Recommended Reading

The 14-page booklet *The Rene Caisse Formula Interview* is an interview of Sheila Snow by Mali Klein in October 1996. The booklet is available for a donation sent to this address:

The Clouds Trust
PO Box 3, Liss,
Hampshire GU33 7XF
United Kingdom

Their website is www.cloudstrust.org

Essiac: A Native Herbal Cancer Remedy, by Cynthia Olsen, et al. (Kali Press, 1998).

For more information go to: http://essiac-info.org/

GERSON THERAPY

The Gerson Therapy consists of diet and detoxification. Dr. Max Gerson, a graduate of the University of Freiburg Medical School in Germany, who fled to the United States in 1936 as a refugee from fascism, developed the therapy.

What to Expect

This controversial diet involves 12 or more glasses daily of freshly pressed juices, prepared hourly from organically grown fruits and vegetables; 3 full vegetarian meals, freshly prepared from organically grown fruits and vegetables; and individual medications. Coffee enemas to induce the liver to release accumulated toxins play an important role in the therapy. If you are going to use the Gerson Therapy, it must be followed *exactly,* with no variation.

Benefits

The Gerson Therapy has benefited some individuals/patients with adenocarcinoma, breast cancer, brain cancer, candida, cataracts, cervical cancer, insomnia, among others, by stimulating the production of natural immune factors.

Recommended Reading

The Gerson Therapy: The Amazing Nutritional Program for Cancer and Other Illnesses, by Charlotte Gerson and Walker Morton, D.P.M. (Kensington, 2001).

Additional Resources

In 1999, the Gerson Institute moved its facilities to Oasis, and this is where Charlotte Gerson is currently working. Diet and nutrition are very important at this facility. The Gerson program is, however, separate from Oasis's program. The Gerson Institute is located at Oasis of Hope Hospital (Contreras Clinic) in Tijuana, Mexico. Call (888) 500-4673 to arrange a phone consultation with a doctor or 011 52 664 631 61 00 if outside the United States.

HOMEOPATHY

Homeopathy is a 200-year-old system of medicine that is based on three principles:

- **Like cures like:** For example, if the symptoms of your cold are similar to poisoning by mercury, then mercury would be your homeopathic remedy.
- **Minimal dose:** The remedy is taken in an extremely dilute form; normally 1 part of the remedy to around 1,000,000,000,000 parts of water.
- **The single remedy:** No matter how many symptoms are experienced, only one remedy is taken, and that remedy will be aimed at all those symptoms.

Homeopathic medicine is a natural pharmaceutical science that uses specific plants, minerals, or animal extracts in very small doses that elicit symptoms in a patient in order to stimulate a person's natural defenses. By causing an overdose of symptoms, the homeopathic treatment actually strengthens a person's healing systems. The remedies given are extremely diluted and encourage the body's own energy to react and repair. Homeopathy treats all symptoms as one, which in practical terms means that it addresses the cause of the illness, not just the symptoms. This often means that symptoms tackled with homeopathy do not recur.

What to Expect

When you first visit a homeopath, you will be asked questions relating to your medical history, your immediate family's medical history, and your lifestyle (your dietary habits, sleep patterns, exercise regimen, and stress levels) to ensure that a holistic approach is taken. The practitioner may also carry out a series of tests, such as checking your glands, breathing, and blood pressure. Your first visit will always be longer than following visits, since the homeopath needs to draw up a full picture of the person being treated. Once the homeopath determines a course of treatment, you will be advised on how and when to take the homeopathic remedies. Professional homeopaths receive national certification (CCH) from the Council of Homeopathic Certification (CHC).

Benefits

Homeopathy is an increasingly popular and accepted, inexpensive, and easy-to-administer treatment. Unlike other medicines, homeopathic medicines usually do not have any adverse side effects. They do not have any chemical action, so they do not have the potential to cause any sustained damage. Homeopathic medicines are very effective in both acute and chronic conditions. Homeopathic medicines are usually dispensed as sweet pills that are very easy to take.

Recommended Reading
The Complete Homeopathy Handbook: A Guide to Everyday Health Care, by Miranda Castro (St. Martin's Press, 1991).

MIND/BODY TECHNIQUES

Mind/body medicine is an approach to healing that uses the power of thoughts and emotions to influence physical health. As Hippocrates once wrote, "The natural healing force within each one of us is the greatest force in getting well." Mind and body techniques can be extremely effective in creating inner calm and coping with the side effects of breast cancer. To relax the mind, women can learn relaxation exercises, meditation, self-hypnosis, imagery, or other skills that can effectively relieve the side effects of breast cancer without the side effects of pharmaceutical approaches. The key to any mind/body technique is to "train" the mind to focus on the body without distraction. It is in this state of "focused concentration" that an individual may be able to change his or her health. The following are some of the most commonly practiced techniques.

Breathwork

Using breath awareness, a simple and natural way to access the inner world of the human psyche can be discovered. Through the process, you can get in touch with and heal suffering caused by unconscious conditioning, unresolved birth trauma, or old emotional wounds, and access altered states of consciousness.

What to Expect
Certified facilitators of breathwork will guide students through different methods of achieving various states of consciousness through evocative music, reciprocating partnerships in breathing sessions, art, focused energy release work, and group sharing. The goals of these exercises are wholeness,

healing, and wisdom. The breathwork experience is, for the most part, internal and largely nonverbal.

Benefits

Breathwork can be an invaluable tool for growth on the spiritual path as a method for personal healing and well-being, particularly in times of stress or recovery. Benefits of breathwork include:

- Anxiety/stress reduction.
- Emotional stability.
- Greater self-image and self-esteem.
- Joy and happiness.
- Inner peace.
- A greater spiritual awareness.

Recommended Reading

The Breathwork Experience: Exploration and Healing in Nonordinary States of Consciousness, by Kylea Taylor (Hanford Mead, 1994).

Energy Healing

Energy healing (also called aura and chakra healing) is one of the most fundamental therapies in the field of alternative medicine and holistic health. It uses spiritual healing methods and energy, color, and light healing techniques to help the patient break free from afflictions and limitations of body, mind, and spirit.

What to Expect

During an energy healing, the healer utilizes a blend of techniques depending on the client's needs. These techniques include, but are not limited to breathwork, visualization, and muscle checking (when resistance is applied to isolated muscles, the physical body will respond with a strong or weak muscle, depending on the flow of energy within the body). During a session, a client lies on a treatment table and is guided in some breathing and visualization to relax. Muscle checking is then used to communicate with the client's body-mind system to obtain information about how energy is being held in the body and where there might be blocks, constrictions, and imbalances. The muscle-checking technique also allows limiting emotions and belief systems to be identified and then released through breath, visualization, and occasionally light hands-on work. Affirmations are subsequently introduced so that the body, mind, emotions and spirit can align with new, empowering energies for a permanent and transformational experience.

Benefits

Energy healing is a holistic, mind-body-spirit system of self-healing. Energy healing can have a significant positive impact on many emotional side effects of breast cancer and its treatment. Many practitioners are able to relieve themselves of trauma and emotional buildup, detoxify the mind, body, and spirit, and increase their spiritual awareness.

Recommended Reading

Quantum-Touch: The Power to Heal, by Richard Gordon and C. Norman Shealy (North Atlantic Books, 1999).

Guided Imagery or Therapeutic Imagery

Guided imagery is the use of pleasant or relaxing images and controlled breathing to calm the mind and body and achieve a state of deep relaxation. This relatively easy method can be learned by anyone. Imagery has been used in addition to conventional therapy in the treatment of cancer and other conditions, in which a patient visualizes disease states being driven out of the body. Therapeutic imagery is currently being used in many cancer resource programs to benefit the women who are receiving services.

What to Expect

This relatively easy method can be learned by anyone, and practiced with the assistance of a therapist, practitioner, friend, or even on your own. The most common exercise in guided imagery involves visualizing a relaxing, pleasing place that makes you feel safe and secure. By imaging details that bring you closer to that place and which describe it, you are able to relax and distract your mind.

Benefits

Imagery is a relaxation technique designed to release brain chemicals that act as your body's natural brain tranquilizers, lowering blood pressure, heart rate, and anxiety levels. Because imagery relaxes the body, doctors specializing in imagery often recommend it for stress-related conditions and for the stressful side effects of treatments, surgery, and disease.

Recommended Reading
Staying Well with Guided Imagery, by Belleruth Naparstek (Warner Books, 1995).

Meditation

Meditation is a globally recognized discipline or practice of contemplation or awareness, but not a treatment in the usual medical sense. Meditation is, however, frequently recommended by mainstream medical practitioners (as well as alternative therapists), because of its healing effects on the central nervous system, heart rate, and muscular tension. The feelings achieved during meditation vary for each person but are generally expressed as feelings of wholeness and complete disconnectedness at the same time. To experience any type or level of meditation takes practice.

What to Expect
People can learn to meditate in a variety of ways. There are many fine self-help books written from a variety of religious and philosophical perspectives that explain the basic techniques of meditation. Most people, however, can benefit from an experienced teacher or spiritual guide. The form of meditation with which most Westerners are familiar involves sitting quietly in a chair or on the floor for a period of time with eyes closed in order to concentrate or focus the mind. There are, however, a variety of approaches to meditation practice including breathing exercises, body scanning, mantras, devotion, visualization, moving meditation, walking meditation, various forms of yoga, and sufi walking. Remember, even a few minutes of meditation can be beneficial.

Benefits
Many women use meditation to reduce stress during or after cancer treatment, to gain concentration and focus, to mentally aid healing, to create self-empowerment and goal fulfillment, or to reach an enlightened spiritual state. It is important to understand that although better health is a

HUMOR/LAUGHTER

The role of humor in healing for patients and survivors of breast cancer is rarely discussed or prescribed by physicians. Fear, sadness, and despondency often produce negative outcome, while a humorous outlook can help in the healing process. Humor is an important and valuable tool to help women redefine the breast and reclaim their bodies psychologically.

Laughter can stimulate endorphins—chemicals that act like opiates in the brain. Writer Norman Cousins discovered that 10 minutes of genuine belly laughter had an anesthetic effect that would give him at least 2 hours of pain-free sleep.

Therapeutically speaking, humor is one of the healthiest and most powerful methods available to help cancer patients gain a new perspective on life's most difficult experiences. In addition, giving oneself time to not think about cancer can be emotionally beneficial.

Recommended Reading

Not Now . . . I'm Having a No Hair Day: Humor and Healing for People with Cancer, by Christine Clifford (Pfeifer-Hamilton, 1996).

frequent side effect of meditation, it is not the goal or focus of meditation practice.

Recommended Reading
Journey into Day: Meditations for New Cancer Patients, by Rusty Freeman (Judson Press, 2000).

Spirituality

Spirituality is the realization of the universality of truth and the experience of bliss. It is an opportunity to realize and become conscious of a Supreme Reality (in some cases, a God), with which or whom we can have a relationship. It is an experience involving an awareness of and relationship with something that transcends your personal self as well as the human order of things. This Supreme Reality can provide an experience of inspiration, joy, security, peace of mind, and guidance that goes beyond what is possible in the absence of the conviction that such a power exists. In reality, religion and spirituality are quite similar. Spirituality is at the core of all religions.

Benefits

A number of studies have associated a deep religious faith with an ability to cope more effectively with cancer, including breast cancer. Researchers at the University of Texas Health Science Center at San Antonio published a study about the impact of deep faith on the condition of women with breast cancer. They found that with a group of Anglo-American patients, "intrinsic religiousness" was a strong predictor of spiritual well-being and hope—both of which are important factors for successfully coping with cancer.

Recommended Reading

Speak the Language of Healing: Living With Breast Cancer Without Going to War, by Susan Kuner, Carol M. Orsborn, Linda Quigley, and Karen L. Stroup (Conari Press, 1999).

NATUROPATHY

More of a philosophical approach to health than a particular form of therapy, naturopathy is a way of treating illnesses that works on the principle that healing depends on the action of natural healing forces present in the human body. Naturopathic medicine offers a wide variety of natural, noninvasive remedies for an array of troubling ailments. Supporters of naturopathy see disease as a disruption of processes that can be healed naturally through diet, herbal remedies, exercise, homeopathy, massage, spinal and soft tissue manipulation, hydrotherapy (use of water to promote healing), counseling, light therapy, and other techniques. Some naturopaths practice Oriental medicine, including acupuncture.

What to Expect

Naturopathic doctors cooperate with all branches of medical science, referring individuals to other practitioners for diagnosis or treatment when appropriate. Naturopathic practitioners range from physicians to massage therapists, and their approach to diagnosis varies accordingly. Among all practitioners, evaluation of diet and lifestyle is considered crucial. However, if your practitioner has a high level of medical expertise, diagnosis may also involve laboratory analysis, allergy tests, X rays, and a physical exam. Naturopaths are not involved in the practice of medicine and do not use drugs or pharmaceuticals. Though few states recognize naturopathy, it is indeed an established course of study. When seeking a naturopathic treatment, you should make sure you choose one certified as a Doctor of Naturopathy (N.D.). Many chiropractors or practitioners of Chinese medicine also practice naturopathy in those states where naturopathic programs are approved.

Benefits

Naturopathy endeavors to cure disease by channeling the body's own natural healing powers. Rejecting synthetic drugs and invasive procedures, it stresses the restorative powers of nature, the search for underlying causes of disease, and the treatment of the whole person. Naturopathy takes the medical motto "First, do no harm" very seriously.

Recommended Reading

How to Prevent and Treat Cancer with Natural Medicine, edited by Michael T. Murray (Riverhead Books, 2002).

Additional resources

The American Association of Naturopathic Physicians
601 Valley Street, Suite 105
Seattle, WA 98109
http://www.naturopathic.org
(206) 298-0125

TRADITIONAL CHINESE MEDICINE

Traditional Chinese medicine (TCM) is a complete medical system that has diagnosed, treated, and prevented illness for over 23 centuries. The practice is based on the belief that opposition is necessary for balance throughout all aspects of life: earth and heaven, winter and summer, night and day, body and mind. Two primary, oppositional components exist: the yin (negative) and yang (positive). Health is a delicate balance, and the goal of TCM is to restore this balance in the body. If a person's life energy, qi, is blocked, the balance between the body's yin and yang disappears and leaves the body vulnerable to disease.

What to Expect

A medical examination can detect imbalances and blocked qi. To determine the pattern of disharmony and suggest an appropriate treatment, the traditional Chinese doctor uses four diagnostic tools: looking, listening and smelling (which in Chinese are the same word), asking, and touching. The doctor asks a variety of questions in order to discover the patient's medical history, lifestyle, and symptoms. Different parts of the patient's body are felt to detect swelling or soreness. The doctor also feels for the patient's pulse at three places on each wrist. Chinese doctors tally 28 different pulse qualities; each one reflects a particular type of imbalance.

TCM doctors rely on exercise techniques such as qigong and tai chi to strengthen and balance qi, and utilize acupuncture, acupressure, and a full herbal pharmacopoeia, with remedies for most ailments, including breast cancer. Chinese herbal teas, philosophy, and relaxation techniques are soothing to many patients with breast cancer, who use them as complementary therapies.

How to Choose a Practitioner

As with practitioners of more generalized CAM, in the United States, TCM practitioners typically specialize in a particular component of TCM, such as acupuncture, herbs, or massage, rather than the entire discipline. The regulation of TCM varies from state to state. Acupuncturists are licensed in many states, and Doctors of Oriental Medicine (O.M.D.) are licensed in some states to prescribe herbal remedies as well as acupuncture treatments.

Mastering the full range of Chinese medicine is a complex process that requires many years of study and practice. However, medical personnel with less training may still be able to perform acupuncture and herbal medicine safely, by working according to protocols designed by TCM practitioners. As you would with any health provider, check into your TCM practitioner's training and background. As always, be sure to work in conjunction with your primary care physician, and notify your doctor of any TCM therapy you are involved with.

Benefits

The various techniques used in traditional Chinese medicine can address a wide range of illnesses, including breast cancer. Chinese massage techniques may utilize the same points as acupuncture to unblock the flow of your qi and to ease the stress and tension that often accompany illness. Generally speaking, Chinese herbs are safer than Western pharmaceuticals and rarely have unpleasant side effects. They can be purchased at an Asian grocery store or Chinese pharmacy and are relatively inexpensive and easy to use.

Recommended Reading
Between Heaven and Earth: A Guide to Chinese Medicine, by Harriet Beinfield and Efrem Korngold (Ballantine Books, 1992).
The Web That Has No Weaver, by Ted Kaptchuk (McGraw-Hill, 2000).

Acupuncture

Acupuncture is an ancient technique in which a skilled practitioner inserts hair-thin needles into specific points on the body to prevent or treat illness. Practiced for over 2,500 years in China, acupuncture is part of the holistic system of traditional Chinese medicine. Acupuncture is a therapy based on the principle that there is an "energetic connection" between the organs of the body and the body surface. When an organ is diseased, the correlating acupuncture points, which are connected by channels that cover the interior and exterior of the body, are often tender to the touch if that organ system is experiencing imbalance. The sufferer sometimes feels the tender spot or spots himself or may only realize they are there when a skilled practitioner presses over the point.

What to Expect
According to the principles of TCM, chi flows through the body via 14 primary meridians or channels. To strengthen the flow of chi, or remove blockages in the meridians, an acupuncturist inserts a number of tiny, sterile, flexible needles just under the skin at certain specific points along the channels. There are hundreds of acupoints along the meridians, which are associated with specific internal organs or organ systems. Generally, 3 to 15 needles will be placed in various locations on the body. (As an admitted needle-phobe, I find acupuncture to be a nearly pain-free procedure.)

Costs vary depending on locale and the practitioners' training and experience, and session lengths depend upon the amount of areas that need to be addressed. It is possible to feel relief after a single session, but follow-up visits may be necessary for maintenance, or for treating intense symptoms. Duration and frequency of acupuncture treatment depends on the ailment and the particular person being treated.

Benefits
Acupuncture is effective for control of pain and of local postoperative swelling, for diminishing tissue swelling, and for minimizing use and side effects of pain-relieving medications. In conjunction with nutritional support, acupuncture is routinely performed in some cancer care facilities.

Recommended Reading
Fundamentals of Chinese Acupuncture, by Nigel Wiseman (Paradigm, 1991).
Grasping the Wind, by Nigel Wiseman and Andy Ellis (Paradigm, 1989).

Chinese Herbs
Chinese herbal medicine is the oldest and most comprehensive form of internal medicine and is one of the main components of TCM. Currently, many Chinese herbal therapies are being studied in conjunction with Western medical treatment for the treatment of cancer, especially for breast cancer. If you have cancer or a serious systemic illness, it is appropriate to consult a licensed practitioner of Chinese herbal therapy to discuss potential uses, since there are over 500 herbs commonly used in traditional Chinese medicine. As with any complementary treatment, consult with your physician regarding dosage and possible side effects before taking any herbal supplements.

In addition to herbs such as garlic, green tea, and maitake that may prevent the spread of cancer, some herbs used to treat the physical and emotional effects of breast cancer include:

- *Black cohosh* treats hot flashes.
- *Echinacea* treats mouth ulcers that occur during chemotherapy.
- *Ginger* relieves nausea and vomiting associated with chemotherapy.
- *Horehound* relieves loss of appetite.
- *Mistletoe* prevents immune suppression (especially during chemotherapy).
- *St. John's wort* relieves pain, treats anxiety and depression, heals and soothes inflamed or irriated skin (especially after radiation), relieves loss of appetite (especially during chemotherapy), and may prevent spread of cancer.

What to Expect

When Chinese herbs are used, generally many are prescribed together for their synergistic effect. Herbal tonics for restoring healthy internal organ function may require weeks of use, whereas herbs for colds and flu can show good results in hours.

Benefits

Traditionally, many herbs were used to treat cancer and enhance immunity, and currently many of these are being studied for their ability to influence our overall immunity.

Qigong

The word qigong is made up of two Chinese words: "qi," meaning "life force energy," and "gong," meaning "work." An ancient Chinese art of self-healing, this exercise system is based on slow, gently flowing movements combined with mental concentration and controlled breathing to enhance overall well-being and healing

What to Expect

Qigong exercises that involve the entire body (arms, legs, shoulders, hips, feet, torso, and so on) are combined with breathing patterns to create movement patterns to manipulate and channel your body's energy, or your qi. It is helpful to learn qigong with an experienced teacher; however, the simple movements can be learned and practiced at home.

Benefits

Qigong's gentle movements and soothing breathing and meditation exercises can aid in relaxation, stress relief, and alleviating the body and mind fatigue often associated with breast cancer treatment. The practice can also bring your entire being closer to balance, harmony, and peace.

Recommended Reading

Qi Gong for Beginners: Eight Easy Movements for Vibrant Health, by Stanley D. Wilson (Sterling, 1997).

Tai Chi

Much like qigong, tai chi is an ancient Chinese form of coordinated body movements focusing on the cultivation of internal energy. Its aim is to harmonize the mind, body, and spirit, promoting both mental and phys-ical well-being through relaxation. When practiced correctly, the move-ments of tai chi appear rhythmical, effortless, and in continuous flow. Unlike most forms of exercise and sport, tai chi does not rely on strength, force, and speed, making it ideal for people of both sexes, young and old alike, whether strong or weak.

What to Expect

Tai chi is learned by doing. It takes about three months to learn the set, and the beginner class format is quite simple. The instructor will demon-strate a move several times, then perform it with the class, and finally watch the students as they repeat it. The exercises can be performed in any com-fortable clothing. Shoes that offer good support and balance, like comfort-able walking shoes or sneakers, are required, but there are no special uniforms.

Benefits

Tai chi is becoming recognized in the medical community as an impor-tant adjunct to conventional treatments for many ailments and diseases, in-cluding breast cancer. Practiced diligently, a student of tai chi will become revitalized, relaxed, tolerant, self-confident, and stronger and healthier in both mind and body.

Recommended Reading

Beginner's Tai Chi Chuan, by Vincent Chu (Unique, 2000).

YOGA

Yoga (from the Sanskrit word for "union" or "oneness") is a personal self-help system of health care and spiritual development. Developed in In-dia, yoga is a psychophysical discipline with roots going back about 5,000 years. Today, most yoga practices in the West focus on the physical postures, called "asanas," breathing exercises, called "pranayama," and meditation, which promote improved physical fitness, mental clarity, greater self-understanding, stress control, and general well-being. Spirituality, however, is a strong underlying theme to most practices. The beauty of yoga is in its versatility, allowing practitioners to focus on the physical, psychological, or spiritual, or a combination of all three.

What to Expect

There are many different forms of yoga, some very rigorous and others meditative and soothing. The following are some popular yoga disciplines:

- Hatha yoga, which incorporates breathing, physical postures, and relaxation and meditation to enhance the union of mind, body, and spirit. Hatha yoga has become popular in the West and is the type of yoga that is frequently taught at yoga studios, health clubs, and recreational facilities.
- Ashtanga yoga (Eightfold Path) involves synchronizing the breath with progressive series of postures—a process producing intense internal heat and a profuse, purifying sweat that detoxifies muscles and organs. This can be very rigorous exercise and women undergoing chemotherapy may not want to take this form of yoga.
- Kundalini yoga, called the "yoga of awareness," is an ancient system of exercise, breath control, and meditation using safe and comprehensive techniques that enhances awareness and increases vitality.
- Kripalu yoga uniquely blends the physical postures of hatha yoga with contemplative meditation. Strong emphasis on breath awareness and breathing techniques is part of the foundation of kripalu yoga.
- Iyengar yoga is an approach to hatha yoga that makes frequent use of props. Objects like blocks, chairs, blankets, and belts are used to help you adjust yourself to the different postures so that you can work in a range of motion that is safe and effective for you. Use of support, force, and resistance from props can allow for a pose with more depth and awareness.

During cancer treatment, particularly chemotherapy, it will be extremely important for you to stay hydrated and not to overexert yourself. Women actively undergoing treatment may wish to choose a more relaxed class that focuses on stretching and posture, tone, and concentration.

You should wear clothing that is easy to move in, such as loose-fitting sweatpants, leggings, T-shirts, tank tops, and so on. Also be aware that yoga is practiced in bare feet; however, if this is absolutely out of the question for you, socks are permissible. Mats and hand towels are usually provided at yoga classes (sometimes for a small fee). Because many others use the mats, you may want to consider purchasing your own personal yoga mat to bring to class for hygienic reasons. Remember to also bring a bottle of water.

Benefits

Many cancer centers and retreat programs for women with breast cancer have yoga classes for their patients as the exercises can have many strengthening and toning physical benefits, and soothing and healing emotional effects.

Recommended Reading

Yoga: The Spirit and Practice of Moving into Stillness, by Erich Schiffmann (Pocket Books, 1996).

16.

INNOVATIVE TREATMENTS & LOW-TOXICITY DRUGS

· ·

INNOVATIVE TREATMENTS

714X (Naessen or Immunostim)

714X is an aqueous solution of camphoriminium chloride and contains ammonium chloride, nitrate, sodium chloride, ethanol, and water. More than 800 cancer patients have received 714X, and it has recently been transferred from experimental to investigational status.

What to Expect

The dose consists of 3 consecutive series of 21 daily injections directly into the lymphatic system. Treatment is stopped for 3 days and continued at the rate of 7 injections per week for a minimum of 2 to 4 months or longer, depending on the response of each individual patient. Treatment is then repeated until the progress of the disease is reversed. An average of 7 to 12 treatment cycles is recommended for metastatic or advanced disease. A healthy diet following holistic nutrition guidelines accompanies the treatment (i.e., no sugar, low fat, no dairy, no pork or beef). Despite decades of use with 714X, no clinical trials have been performed; therefore, little is known about potential risks.

Benefits

Supporters claim that 714X acts as an immune enhancer or booster to stimulate the body's ability to regain balance; the treatment does not attack the cancer cell directly but stabilizes the human organism's natural defenses. There are many anecdotal reports of successful outcomes among patients who have used 714X, although there are no formal clinical studies, animal studies, or cell system studies documenting its effectiveness.

Additional Resources
Cose, Inc.
5270 rue Fontain
Rock Forest, Quebec
Canada J1N 2B6
(819) 564-7883

Antineoplastons

Antineoplastons are naturally occurring peptides. They were originally isolated from human blood and urine by Stanislaw Burzynski, M.D., Ph.D., who claims they can "reprogram" cancerous cells to behave like "normal" cells again. The Burzynski Research Institute is currently conducting clinical trials of antineoplastons.

What to Expect

Burzynski's therapies are delivered intravenously through a catheter inserted in a central venous line. A pump infuses the medications at scheduled intervals. The dose and dosing schedule depend on the type of cancer. The pump and the therapy bags are small and light enough to be carried around by a young child. Now many patients take only capsules or tablets without intravenous injections. The major disadvantages of the treatment are that it is quite expensive and that patients have to travel to Dr. Burzynski's clinic in Houston, Texas, to receive the treatment.

Benefits

The success of antineoplaston treatments has been highly controversial; the American Cancer Society reports that they have no reliable evidence of the objective benefits of antineoplastons. Burzynski reported that the antineoplaston peptides are essentially nontoxic and that preliminary clinical results indicated tumor responses (shrinkages) in a number of difficult cases, most of which involved subjects who had exhausted conventional treatments. This therapy has most often been used for people with gliomas. Dr. Burzynski has been funded for some clinical trials in this area.

Additional Resources
The Burzynski Clinic
9432 Old Katy Road, Suite 200
Houston, TX 77055
www.cancermed.com
(713) 335-5697

Enzyme Therapy

Each of the body's thousands of different enzymes aid in specific chemical reactions in the body. Deficiencies or overabundance of particular enzymes in the bloodstream can indicate that the body is reacting to a particular disease or ailment. When the body is unable to produce sufficient quantities of its own enzymes, enzyme replacement therapy is often used to treat the affected enzyme group. Enzymes can be taken orally or by injection, usually taken between meals so they are not used up during the digestion of mealtime foods.

What to Expect
For genuine cases of enzyme deficiency, verified by blood tests and assessment of digestive status, doctors prescribe supplements such as Donnazyme, Cotazyme, Creon, Pancrease, Ultrase, and Zymase. Enzyme products promoted for other disorders are typically sold as dietary supplements.

Benefits
It is theorized that with solid tumors, enzyme therapy slowly works to degrade the cell walls of cancer cells, reducing growth and making other treatments more effective.

Recommended Reading
The Complete Book of Enzyme Therapy, by Anthony Cichoke (Avery, 1998).

Additional Resources
Digestive Disease National Coalition (DDNC)
711 Second Street NE, Suite 200

Washington, DC 20002
(202) 544-7497

The Gonzalez Protocol

The Gonzalez Protocol is a complicated regimen that includes taking oral pancreatic enzymes, coffee enemas, and more than 150 pills daily, including vitamins, minerals, papaya extract, and animal glandular extracts. It is used to treat pancreatic cancer and possibly other cancers. The National Institute of Health's National Center for Complementary and Alternative Medicine (NCCAM) is currently funding the Gonzalez Protocol Trial, a 5-year clinical study.

What to Expect

The Gonzalez Protocol is a very demanding regimen that should only be undertaken under a doctor's strict supervision, because of the potentially toxic effects of combining many different supplements.

Benefits

One of the attractive points of this therapy is the cost. The total cost of the program runs about $5,000 to $6,000 per year. Supplements constitute 70 to 80 percent of the cost. There is generally no hospitalization involved.

Additional Resources

For information about patient entry into the trial, contact:

Michelle Gabay, R.N.
NewYork-Presbyterian: The University Hospitals of Columbia and Cornell
(212) 305-9468

Hoxsey Therapy

Hoxsey is an herbal concoction composed of pokeroot, burdock root, barberry root, buckthorn bark, and stillinga root. Harry M. Hoxsey said he obtained it from his grandfather, a farmer who observed one of his horses apparently cure itself of cancer by instinctively eating certain plants.

What to Expect

Hoxsey is administered in two forms. One is taken orally and the other is a salve (containing bloodroot), which, if the tumor is on or close to the surface of the skin, is applied topically.

Benefits

Scientific research has identified antitumor activity of one sort or another in all but three of Hoxsey's plants, one of them (*Rhamnus purshiana*) containing the anthraquinone glycoside structure now recognized as predictive of antitumor properties.

Recommended Reading

When Healing Becomes a Crime: The Amazing Story of the Hoxsey Cancer Clinics and the Return of Alternative Therapies, by Kenny Ausubel (Healing Arts Press, 2000).

Additional Resources

Bio-Medical Center
PO Box 727
615 General Ferreira, Colonia Juarez
Tijuana, B.C.
Mexico

Newcastle Disease Virus (MTH-68)

This is a treatment that involves deliberately infecting patients with the virus that causes Newcastle disease (NDV) in poultry. Dr. Ralph Moss, one of the most prestigious investigators in the area of alternative medicine, has been involved in the research of NDV.

What to Expect

MTH-68 is a carefully crafted variant on the NDV virus vaccine. It is a biological product derived from the "H" strain of the attenuated (somewhat weakened) NDV vaccine. The final product is a purified version of the virus, which has been used in human cancer patients. Currently, the medicine is being taken either nasally as a spray or drip, or rectally as a suppository. The medicine comes in a powder form, which is mixed with a saline solution before one takes it. It takes only minutes to administer.

Benefits

For three decades, several dozen papers have shown the effectiveness of the NCV in the treatment of cancer. In the medical literature that documented its anticancer activity, the *Journal of the National Cancer Institute* indicates: "We are entering a new age of viral therapeutics for human cancer." This treatment is almost completely lacking in side effects in humans, with fevers being the most commonly reported.

Laetrile (Amygdalin)

When the natural substance called amygdalin is purified and concentrated for use in cancer therapy, it is called laetrile. Amygdalin is extracted from apricot seeds and prepared in both tablet and injectable form. It is a carcinogenic compound. In 1977, a synthesized version was developed by an FDA–Johns Hopkins team and was given the name laetrile. Today about 21 states permit the importing and medical use of laetrile in cancer treatment.

What to Expect

Laetrile is commonly given intravenously over a period of time and then orally as maintenance therapy (treatment given to help extend the benefit of previous therapy). When taken intravenously, laetrile is converted by cancer cell enzymes into cyanide, which then kills the cell. *Never take large amounts of laetrile orally.*

Benefits

Laetrile is a hydrocyanic acid, which supporters claim kills cancer cells.

Coley's Toxins (Mixed Bacterial Vaccine or MBV)

Coley's Toxins are a treatment for cancer devised by Dr. William Coley, a New York surgeon. After experimentation, he developed a serum that came to be known as Coley's Toxins, a mixture of heat-killed bacteria. Coley gradually adjusted the doses until he got a good response—fever, rash, chills, shakes, and other symptoms, which are referred to as the "cytokine flu."

What to Expect

The toxins are injected into the patient, either directly into or around the tumors.

Benefits

The toxins were said to be successful with sarcomas (soft-tissue cancers), and some current experts have speculated that their beneficial effects may extend to all cancers that originate in mesodermal tissue (including kidney and ovarian cancer).

Additional Resources
Waisbren Clinic
Burton A. Waisbren, Sr., M.D., F.A.C.P.
2315 N. Lake Drive
Room 815, Seton Tower
Milwaukee, WI 53211
(414) 272-1929

Cancer Research Institute
681 Fifth Avenue
New York, NY 10022
(800) 223-7874, or (800) 522-5022 in New York
Mrs. Nauts (Coley's daughter), who is the director of communications for CRI, can be reached at 1225 Park Avenue, New York, NY 10128, (212) 722-8547.

Psychotherapy

A psychotherapist is a counselor or support person who helps people with their emotional, social, and mental processes. Usually, a psychotherapist has a master's-level degree in either social work or psychology and is generally licensed or certified by the state licensing board. Talking with a trained therapist about life events may be focused on coping with illness and changes associated with it. It can also focus on personal growth and on increasing joy in living.

How do you know if psychotherapy might be useful for you? Some possible reasons are when you:

- Feel depressed and hopeless, yet sense you have exhausted your family and personal support resources.
- Are overwhelmed with fears and worries.
- Can't make decisions.

- Worry excessively (your call) about your children, marriage, job, and yourself.
- Have thoughts of suicide.
- Have difficulty dealing with the thought of recurrence and/or death to the point that your life seems stalled.
- Need help figuring out the direction and meaning of your life.

What to Expect

The role of the therapist is to stabilize and facilitate treatment so that a person can move back to a baseline level of functioning. Going to a therapist does not mean you are emotionally sick or mentally weak—it is not about blame. A good therapist is trained to ask the right questions, to foster decision-making skills, and to point out options you might overlook. Once life circumstances have become more settled, a therapist can help to explore issues of meaning and direction in life, when old perspectives no longer seem to fit. Therapists may be involved in directing patients back to their physicians if medication is necessary.

Benefits

Psychotherapy positively affects physical health and for many is a helpful supplement to conventional cancer therapies. Patients with breast cancer benefit from psychosocial support during treatment, particularly in alleviating anxiety and depression and increasing knowledge. Patients experience significant improvement in mood, coping, and both physical and functional adjustment.

Cellular Therapy

Cellular therapy refers to various procedures in which processed tissue from animal embryos, fetuses, or organs is injected or taken by mouth. Cellular therapy, as practiced today, was developed in the early 1930s by the Swiss physician Paul Niehans. It soon became popular with celebrities as a means of rejuvenation. Cellular therapy is also called live cell therapy, cellular suspensions, glandular therapy, fresh cell therapy, siccacell therapy, embryonic cell therapy, and organotherapy. Products are obtained from specific organs or tissues said to correspond with the unhealthy organs or tissues of the recipient. Federal agencies in the United States and Germany have taken several actions to impede the marketing of cellular therapy.

What to Expect

Live cell therapy using animal cells can be dangerous as well as ineffective, because injections of animal cells can spread viral disease and trigger severe allergic reactions. During the 1980s, cases were reported of allergic reactions, brain and nerve damage, immune complex vasculitis, and a blistering skin disease resembling bullous pemphigoid. In 1984, the FDA banned importation into the United States of all cellular powders and extracts intended for injection.

Benefits

Supporters claim that cellular therapy can help build the immune system and help patients with Down's syndrome, Alzheimer's disease, epilepsy, AIDS, cancer, and many other diseases.

Recommended Reading

Cell Therapy, by Yasuo Ikeda, J. Hata, S. Koyasu, and Y. Kawakami (Springer Verlag, 2002). *Note:* This book is very expensive.

LOW-TOXICITY DRUGS

Benzaldehyde

Benzaldehyde, chemically related to benzene, is a colorless oily liquid used as a flavoring agent and to make dyes, perfumes, and pharmaceuticals. It is administered intravenously.

Benefits

Benzaldehyde, also present in burdock, has been shown to have significant anticancer effects in humans. There have been several studies showing antitumor activity from burdock in animal systems.

Gossypol

Gossypol is a natural toxin present in the cotton plant that protects it from insect damage. While it is mostly harvested for fabric, studies show cotton may hold compounds to help fight breast cancer.

Benefits

Supporters claim that gossypol can slow tumor growth. There is no current evidence of this.

Iscador

Iscador is the trade name of the most commonly available brand of an extract of a European species of mistletoe. This variety of mistletoe differs from the North American species. Iscador has been used as an injection before surgery for cancers of the cervix, ovary, breast, stomach, colon, and lung. There are no serious side effects.

Benefits

Iscador has been used in many thousands of cancer patients over a period of at least 70 years. There are anecdotal reports of improved immune function, quality of life, and survival, but no basis for the widespread use of mistletoe preparations.

Recommended Reading

Iscador: Mistletoe in Cancer Therapy, edited by Christine Murphy (Lantern Books, 2001).

Suramin

A drug used to treat bacterial and parasitic infections, suramin is also being studied in the treatment of cancer. Suramin is administered intravenously, sometimes in conjunction with radiation therapy. Possible side effects include a decrease in white and red blood cell and platelet count, a decrease in kidney function, nausea, vomiting or diarrhea, weakness, numbness, mouth sores, blood clots, and rashes.

Benefits

Suramin is being investigated for antitumor qualities, and trials suggest that the agent may help control the growth of the cancer. The most commonly reported benefit is pain reduction.

PART III

Guide to Breast Cancer-Related Drugs

This listing includes drugs typically used to treat breast cancer, including brand and generic names, uses, and common side effects. New breast cancer drugs are frequently introduced to the market, so please be sure to consult with your health professional for the most up-to-date information and options.

ADRIAMYCIN

Generic name: doxorubicin hydrochloride.

Use: Adriamycin is a chemotherapy drug commonly used to treat breast cancer and other cancers. Adriamycin first disrupts, then destroys the growth of cancer cells. It is usually administered intravenously (through the vein).

Possible side effects: Decreased white blood cell count with increased risk of infection, decreased platelet count with increased risk of bleeding, loss of appetite, darkening of nail beds and skin creases of hands, hair loss, nausea and vomiting, and mouth sores.

AREDIA

Generic name: pamidronate disodium.

Use: Aredia is used in patients with breast cancer or multiple myloma whose disease has spread to the bones. Although Aredia is given by intravenous injection, it isn't a form of chemotherapy. Aredia can decrease bone pain in some breast cancer and multiple myeloma patients.

Possible side effects: Some Aredia patients may experience fever, fatigue, nausea, vomiting, bone pain, and lack of appetite, which pass in a few days, and anemia. Your doctor can recommend a mild pain reliever that may help prevent these symptoms or relieve them if they occur. You should talk to your doctor if you experience high temperature, redness, swelling, or pain at the site where Aredia is infused, tiredness, nausea, lack of appetite, or muscle twitching. Your doctor will be checking your blood routinely for anemia and other possible side effects and will be watching your response to this medication.

ARIMIDEX

Generic name: anastrozole.

Use: Arimidex is used for the initial treatment of hormone receptor–positive or hormone receptor–unknown locally advanced or metastatic breast cancer in postmenopausal women. It works best when the tumor is estrogen receptor–positive. Arimidex belongs to a group of medicines called aromatase inhibitors, which work by blocking aromatase, an enzyme needed to make estrogen in postmenopausal women. Estrogens may cause the growth of some types of breast tumors.

Possible side effects: Hot flashes, nausea, decreased energy and weakness, pain, back pain, bone pain, increased cough, mild diarrhea, increased or decreased appetite, temporary hair thinning, vaginal dryness, and joint pain/stiffness.

AROMASIN

Generic name: exemestane.

Use: Aromasin was approved by the FDA in 1999 to treat metastatic breast cancer in postmenopausal women. Aromasin works by binding to the body's aromatase enzyme, an enzyme responsible for producing the hormone estrogen. Many breast cancer cells depend on estrogen to grow and multiply quickly. Once Aromasin has binded to the aromatase enzyme, it cannot produce estrogen and thereby prevents cancer cells from growing. Aromasin is usually taken orally in pill form.

Possible side effects: Hot flashes, nausea, fatigue, increased sweating, and increased appetite.

CISPLATIN

Generic name: plastinol.

Use: Cisplatin is a chemotherapy that is given as an infusion (drip) into the vein through a cannula (a fine tube inserted into the vein). It may also be given through a central line, which is inserted under the skin into a vein near the collarbone.

Possible side effects: Nausea and vomiting are common side effects. Your kidneys may also be mildly affected. Usually when the kidneys are affected you will not experience any symptoms, but in extreme cases the kidneys can be permanently damaged unless treatment is stopped.

CYTOXAN

Generic name: cyclophosphamide.

Use: Cytoxan is a chemotherapy drug commonly used to treat breast cancer and other cancers. Like Adriamycin, Cytoxan first disrupts cancer cells, then destroys them. Cytoxan is taken in tablets by mouth or intravenously.

Possible side effects: Nausea; vomiting; hair thinning or loss; bruising or bleeding; increased general weakness and fatigue; more frequent urination with a greater amount of urine; red coloration to urine; stomach irritation, such as indigestion or heartburn; flushing of the face, neck, and chest; feeling warm or cool; rash and sore throat; blisters in the mouth; decreased white blood count; and increased risk of infection.

DOXIL

Generic name: liposomal doxorobicin.

Use: Doxil is a type of cancer chemotherapy used for treating Kaposi's sarcoma and breast cancer. Doxil is given intraveneously, usually in a hospital or clinic. Doxil interferes with the growth of rapidly growing cells, like cancer cells, and eventually causes cell death. Doxil is used alone or in combination with other cancer chemotherapy agents. Liposomal doxorubicin is a special form of doxorubicin, which may have fewer side effects.

Possible side effects: Diarrhea, facial flushing, hair loss, heartburn, nail discoloration or damage, nausea, red color in urine (may appear for 1 to 2 days after treatment), and red or watery eyes.

ELLENCE

Generic name: epirubicin hydrochloride.

Use: Ellence was approved by the FDA in 1999 to treat early-stage breast cancer after breast surgery in patients whose cancer has spread to the axillary (underarm) lymph nodes. Ellence is given intravenously in combination with two other chemotherapy drugs, cyclophosphamide and fluorouracil.

Possible side effects: Nausea, vomiting, diarrhea, inflammation of the mouth (stomatitis), hair loss, and reduction in white blood cells (myelosuppression).

EPOGEN

Generic name: epoetin alfa.

Use: Epogen is a growth factor that promotes the red blood cell count and reduces the need for transfusions. It may be given intravenously or may also be injected under the skin (subcutaneously). Subcutaneous injections may be given by medical staff or, with appropriate training, may be self-administered by the patient. You and your doctor will decide the best method for you.

Possible side effects: Patients have reported an increase in blood pressure, headache, irregular heartbeat, nausea/vomiting, blockage of blood flow in the access (surgical opening for dialysis tubing), shortness of breath, diarrhea, and increased potassium levels.

EVISTA

Generic name: raloxifene.

Use: The drug Evista is similar to tamoxifen (Nolvadex) in that it acts like estrogen on the bones but not on the breast or uterus. Evista is neither an estrogen nor a hormone, but a SERM (selective estrogen receptor modulator); SERMs appear to block the effects of estrogen that may promote breast cancer, but these drugs act like estrogen in the bones, building them and helping to prevent osteoporosis. Evista can be taken at any time of day, with or without food (may be taken along with a calcium supplement and/or vitamin D), as your doctor prescribes.

Possible side effects: Evista cannot be taken if you are or can become pregnant, are nursing, have severe liver problems, or have had blood clots that required a doctor's treatment. An infrequent side effect of Evista is blood clots in the veins, and the most common side effects include hot flashes and leg cramps.

FARESTON

Generic name: toremifene.

Use: Similar to tamoxifen, Fareston is an antiestrogen SERM that binds to estrogen receptors on breast cancer cells, preventing the cells from growing and dividing.

Possible side effects: Hot flashes, nausea, weight gain, allergic reactions (such as skin rashes), and headache.

FEMARA

Generic name: letrozole.

Use: Femara was approved by the FDA in 1997 to help treat advanced metastatic breast cancer in women whose breast cancer tumors have not responded well to tamoxifen. Femara is an aromatase inhibitor, which in postmenopausal women works by reducing the total amount of estrogen in the body, limiting the amount of estrogen that can affect breast cancer cells.

Possible side effects: Musculoskeletal pain (pain in the skeleton or legs, arms, or back), nausea, headache, joint pain, fatigue, and difficulty breathing.

5-FU

Generic name: fluorouracil.

Use: 5-FU is one of the oldest chemotherapy drugs and has been used for decades. It is a clear and colorless liquid that may be given as a continuous intravenous infusion over 4 to 5 days, or given on a scheduled basis, (e.g., once a week, or once every 3 to 4 weeks, etc.). It is also available in a cream form for treatment of skin cancer.

Possible side effects: The degree and severity of the side effects depend on the amount and schedule of the administration of 5-FU. The most common side effects include soreness of the mouth, difficulty swallowing, diarrhea, stomach pain, low white blood cell counts, low platelet counts, anemia, and sensitive skin (to sun exposure).

GEMZAR

Generic name: gemcitabine hydrochloride.

Use: Gemzar is a chemotherapy drug that is used to treat certain types of cancer. Gemzar is administered intravenously, in a doctor's office, clinic, or hospital, and usually does not require an overnight hospital stay. The length of your treatment may be longer if your doctor is administering other drugs or fluids at the same time. You will generally receive Gemzar once a week for 2 or 3 weeks in a row, followed by a week without treatment. This constitutes one cycle. The number of cycles you receive will also depend on your individual treatment plan. However, most patients receiving Gemzar as their initial therapy get between 4 and 6 cycles of therapy.

Possible side effects: Some patients receiving Gemzar therapy may experience side effects that may interfere with their daily routine. Usually, this is most likely to occur on the day of treatment, or for a day or so following a treatment. The most common side effects of Gemzar include low blood counts; nausea and vomiting; flulike symptoms; swelling, generally in one or both arms or legs; rash, usually mild to moderate, on the extremeties or torso that may or may not be itchy; hair loss (alopecia); and numbness or tingling in the fingers or toes (neurotoxicity).

HERCEPTIN

Generic name: trastuzumab.

Use: Herceptin is FDA approved to treat metastatic breast cancer in women who overexpress the HER2 gene. HER2 (also written HER2/neu) is a growth factor found on the surface of cells that plays a key role in regulating cell growth. Some women are born with or experience a mutation of the HER2 gene during their lifetime, and so extra HER2 receptors may be produced. This overexpression of HER2 causes cells to grow, divide, and multiply more rapidly than normal and may lead to breast cancer. Women who overexpress the HER2 gene tend to have aggressive breast cancers that spread quickly to other regions of the body. Herceptin is also sometimes given to patients who overexpress the HER+++ gene.

Herceptin seeks out HER2 and attaches itself to the protein receptor on the surface of cells. By binding to the cells, Herceptin has been shown to slow the growth and spread of tumors that have an overabundance of HER2 protein receptors. Herceptin is usually given intravenously in an outpatient clinical setting.

Possible side effects: Weakening of the heart muscle, reduction of white blood cells (leukopenia or neutropenia), diarrhea, anemia (a decreased number of red blood cells and a reduced volume of hemoglobin, the protein within red blood cells that carries oxygen), and abdominal pain or infection.

LEUKINE

Generic name: sargramostim.

Use: Leukine is a man-made form of a protein called a growth factor, which is normally produced in your body. This growth factor helps to increase the number and function of your white blood cells. White blood cells, which are made in your bone marrow, fight infections. Leukine is used to help your bone marrow make more white blood cells. Depending on your treatment, Leukine may be given subcutaneously by injection directly beneath the skin, or by slow intravenous infusion, through a needle or catheter placed in one of your veins.

Possible side effects: Some patients taking Leukine may experience side effects, most of which are mild to moderate. Some common side effects may include bone pain, a slight temperature elevation (usually less than 100.5°F or 38°C) for a short period of time after the injection, and swelling, redness, and/or discomfort at the injection site. These skin reactions may occur simply because cells of the immune system are drawn to the injection site.

MEGACE

Generic name: megestrol.

Use: Megace is used to treat advanced breast cancer, typically in women who do not respond well or become resistant to tamoxifen. Megace is a synthetic form of the hormone progesterone. Progesterone is normally secreted by the corpus luteum of the ovary and by the placenta, and acts to prepare the uterus for implantation of the fertilized ovum, to maintain pregnancy, and to promote development of secondary sexual characteristics. Progesterone also counteracts some of the negative effects of estrogen (many breast cancers depend on estrogen to grow and reproduce). In addition to treating advanced breast cancer, Megace may also be used to treat advanced stages of endometrial cancer (cancer of the uterine lining) or to increase appetite in HIV patients. It can also be effective in controlling hot flashes and vaginal bleeding problems in breast cancer patients.

Possible side effects: Because Megace is considered nontoxic, there are few documented side effects associated with the drug. The most common side effect is fluid retention.

NAVELBINE

Generic name: vinorelbine tartrate.

Use: Navelbine is a chemotherapy drug that is given as a treatment for some types of cancer. Navelbine, when prepared for use, becomes a clear, colorless liquid, and is given by injection into a vein (intravenously) or as an infusion through a fine tube (cannula) inserted into a vein (intravenously) via a drip over a short period of time. It may also be given through a central line, which is inserted into a vein near the collarbone. Navelbine is normally given once a week.

Possible side effects: Decreased white blood cell counts, injection site reactions, constipation, nausea or vomiting, reduced kidney function, neurological problems (numbness, tingling, or weakness), hearing problems, hair loss (alopecia), and fatigue/tiredness.

NEUPOGEN

Generic name: filgrastim.

Use: Neupogen stimulates the production of infection-fighting white blood cells. Neupogen is an injectable prescription treatment that stimulates the bone marrow to make more infection-fighting white blood cells called neutrophils—exactly as your own body does when you're healthy.

Possible side effects: With Neupogen, you may experience some side effects. Bone pain is a reported side effect, and in most cases can be managed with nonnarcotic analgesics such as acetaminophen.

NOVANTRONE

Generic name: mitoxantrone.

Use: Novantrone is a cytotoxic agent belonging to a group of compounds called anticancer agents. Novantrone works in three different ways to kill cancer cells:

1. It binds to an enzyme that normally allows the unraveling of DNA. When Novantrone combines with both the enzyme and DNA, the resulting complex is stable and prevents the cell from continuing through the reproduction process.
2. It forms chemical bonds between the two chains that make up a strand of DNA, inhibiting cell reproduction.
3. It forms bonds from one strand of DNA to a different DNA strand, interfering with the reproduction of the cell.

Novantrone is given by intravenous infusion after being diluted with an appropriate solution.

Possible side effects: Decrease in white blood cells and platelets, mild to moderate nausea and vomiting, diarrhea, headache, sore mouth, stomach pain or discomfort pain, swelling, redness or irritation at the injection site, unusual bleeding or bruising, fever, chill, sore throat, cough (flu symptoms), hair loss, chest pain or discomfort, difficulty breathing, wheezing, fast or irregular heartbeat, swollen feet or ankles, a blue-green color of the urine for 24 hours afterward, a temporary bluish color to the whites of the eyes. Novantrone may cause your white blood cell count to go down, which increases your chance of getting an infection. In addition, Novantrone may cause your platelet count to go down, which increases your chance of bleeding.

ONCOVIN

Generic name: vincristine.

Use: Oncovin is one of the older chemotherapy drugs and has been used for many years. When prepared for use, it becomes a clear and colorless liquid and is given by intravenous route only. Oncovin is normally given once a week.

Possible side effects: Low platelet count, anemia, hair loss, bowel paralysis, diarrhea, nerve damage, damage to the veins (it can cause redness and irritation at the site of injection, despite proper injection), and severe damage to the tissues, if liquid leaks from the injection site (extravasation).

OXYCONTIN

Generic name: oxycodone hydrochloride
Use: Oxycontin is used to relieve moderate to severe pain.
Possible side effects: Although side effects from Oxycontin are not common, they can occur. Tell your doctor if any of the following symptoms are severe or do not go away: upset stomach, constipation, or dry mouth. If you experience any of the following symptoms, call your doctor immediately: rapid or slow heartbeat, trouble breathing, hives, skin rash, hallucinations, yellowing of the skin or eyes, headache, or vomiting.

ROXICODONE

Generic name: roxicodone.
Use: Roxicodone is in a class of drugs called narcotic analgesics and is used to treat moderate to severe pain. Roxicodone is habit-forming and should be used only under close supervision, especially if you have an alcohol or drug addiction. Take Roxicodone exactly as directed by your doctor. Do not stop taking Roxicodone suddenly if you have been taking it continuously for more than 5 to 7 days. Stopping suddenly could cause withdrawal symptoms and make you very uncomfortable. Your doctor may want to gradually reduce your dose.

Possible side effects: If you experience any of the following serious side effects, stop taking Roxicodone and seek emergency medical attention: an allergic reaction (difficulty breathing; closing of your throat; swelling of your lips, tongue, or face; or hives); slow, weak breathing; seizures; cold, clammy skin; severe weakness or dizziness; or unconsciousness.

Other less serious side effects may be more likely to occur. Continue to take Roxicodone and talk to your doctor if you experience: constipation;

dry mouth; nausea, vomiting, or decreased appetite; dizziness, tiredness, or lightheadedness; muscle twitches; sweating; itching; decreased urination; or decreased sex drive. Roxicodone will cause drowsiness and fatigue. Avoid alcohol, sleeping pills, antihistamines, sedatives, and tranquilizers except under the supervision of your doctor. These may also make you drowsy. Roxicodone will also cause constipation. Drink plenty of water (6 to 8 full glasses a day) to reduce this side effect. Increasing the amount of fiber in your diet can also help to alleviate constipation.

TAMOXIFEN

Brand name: Nolvadex.

Use: Tamoxifen has been the most commonly prescribed drug to treat breast cancer since its approval by the FDA in the 1970s. Tamoxifen is an antiestrogen and works by competing with the hormone estrogen to bind to estrogen receptors in breast cancer cells. By blocking estrogen in the breast, tamoxifen helps slow the growth and reproduction of breast cancer cells. In 1998, tamoxifen became the first drug to be approved by the FDA to prevent breast cancer after research showed it reduced the chances of developing breast cancer by 50 percent in women at high risk for the disease. Tamoxifen is taken orally in pill form and is a SERM.

Possible side effects: The most common side effect is hot flashes similar to those experienced during menopause. Tamoxifen may induce menopause in women who are close to menopause; however, it rarely does in young women. Other common side effects include vaginal dryness, irregular periods, and weight gain. Women taking tamoxifen may be at slightly increased risk of developing cataracts. Many experts believe tamoxifen may increase the risk of uterine cancer. All women using tamoxifen should have regular gynecological exams and notify their gynecologist of their use of this medication.

TAXOL

Generic name: paclitaxel.

Use: Taxol was first approved by the FDA in 1992 to treat metastatic breast cancer. In 1999, the FDA also approved Taxol to treat early-stage breast cancer in patients who have already received chemotherapy with the drug doxorubicin. Taxol is called a mitotic inhibitor because it interferes with cells during mitosis (cell division). Taxol is usually given intravenously (through the vein).

Possible side effects: Reduced white blood cell count (myelosuppression), hair loss (alopecia), and numbness in the extremities (peripheral neuropathy).

TAXOTERE

Generic name: docetaxel.

Use: Taxotere is a cancer drug that resembles Taxol in chemical structure. Taxotere was approved by the FDA in 1996 to treat metastatic breast cancer in patients who have not responded well to chemotherapy with the drug Adriamycin. In 1998, Taxotere was also approved by the FDA to treat breast cancer that has spread into other areas of the breast or to other parts of the body after treatment with standard chemotherapy. Taxotere inhibits the division of breast cancer cells by acting on the cell's internal skeleton. The drug is usually given intravenously (through the vein).

Possible side effects: Decrease in white blood cells (leukopenia), fever (often a warning sign of infection), fluid retention, allergic reactions, and hair loss. Because the side effects of Taxotere can be bothersome, many physicians will prescribe additional drugs to help counter these effects. For example, dexamethasone is commonly used to prevent fluid retention while on Taxotere.

WELLCOVORIN

Generic name: leucovorin.

Use: Wellcovorin helps to prevent or treat some of the harmful effects of certain medicines, including methotrexate. Wellcovorin can also treat certain kinds of anemia (low blood counts). Wellcovorin may also be given with the chemotherapy medicine 5-fluorouracil (5-FU) to treat colon cancer. Generic leucovorin injections are available. Wellcovorin is for injection into a muscle or for slow injection into a vein. It is given by a health care professional in a hospital or clinic setting.

Possible side effects: Wellcovorin has few side effects; they include: difficulty breathing and skin rash or itching. If you receive Wellcovorin with 5-FU, you may experience more side effects due to the 5-FU. Check with your health care professional if you notice diarrhea or mouth sores that do not get better or that get worse.

XELODA

Generic name: capecitabine.
Use: Xeloda is an oral medication (an oral form of 5-FU) that is used to treat breast cancer that has spread to other parts of the body and has not responded to treatment with certain other medicines. These medicines include paclitaxel (Taxol) and anthracycline-containing therapy such as Adriamycin and Doxil. Xeloda is converted in the body into the substance 5-fluorouracil. In some patients with colon, rectum, or breast cancer, this substance stops cancer cells from growing and decreases the size of the tumor.

Possible side effects: Diarrhea, nausea, vomiting, stomatitis (sores in mouth and throat), abdominal (stomach area) pain, upset stomach, constipation, loss of appetite, and dehydration (these side effects are more common in patients age 80 and older), hand-and-foot syndrome (palms of the hands or soles of the feet tingle or become numb, painful, swollen, or red), rash, dry, itchy, or discolored skin, nail problems, hair loss, tiredness, weakness, dizziness, headache, fever, pain (including chest, back, joint, and muscle pain), trouble sleeping, and taste problems.

Note: These side effects may differ when taking Xeloda in combination with Taxotere. Please consult your doctor for possible side effects that may be caused by taking Xeloda with Taxotere.

ZINECARD

Generic name: dextrazoxane.
Use: Zinecard is taken to reduce the risk of heart damage from Adriamycin (doxorubicin hydrochloride). The danger of heart damage (cardiotoxicity) is one factor that limits the maximum dose of Adriamycin in women with advanced breast cancer. It is not recommended for use with

initial Adriamycin therapy, since it can increase bone marrow suppression caused by chemotherapeutic agents and may interfere with initial antitumor effectiveness of the Adriamycin.

Possible side effects: Pain at site of injection.

ZOLADEX

Generic name: goserelin acetate.

Use: Zoladex is FDA approved to treat advanced breast cancer and prostate cancer. Zoladex works by blocking estrogen from breast cancer cells (and blocking testosterone in men), thereby starving these cells. The drug is typically given by injection under the skin (subcutaneously). Zoladex is a systemic treatment; it cannot distinguish between normal cells and cancer cells; therefore, a variety of side effects are possible.

Possible side effects: Hot flashes, decreased sexual desire, absence of menstruation, vaginal dryness, and breast swelling or tenderness.

The following drugs are not breast cancer–specific drugs but are included as they are frequently prescribed for breast cancer patients.

DECADRON (STEROID)

Generic name: dexamethasone.

Use: Decadron is a steroid that is used in a variety of situations in cancer patients. It comes in intravenous as well as oral tablet forms. Intravenous form is used for immediate action and results, and tablets are used to maintain the effect of Decadron.

- *Antinausea and vomiting:* One dose of Decadron is used prior to chemotherapy, normally along with Zofran, and is given intravenously.
- *Anti-inflammatory:* Decadron is also used in patients who suffer from brain metastasis or spinal cord compression. In these situations, Decadron reduces the swelling of the normal tissues around the cancer site and helps in controlling the symptoms.

Possible side effects: Irritation of stomach, stomach ulcer (most steroids are given with an antiulcer medicine), high blood sugar, high blood pressure, osteoporosis, and fluid retention.

KYTRIL (ANTINAUSEA)

Generic name: granisetron hydrochloride.
Use: Kytril injection is an antinauseant and antiemetic agent. It is administered intravenously within 30 minutes before initiation of chemotherapy, and only on the day(s) chemotherapy is given.
Possible side effects: Headache, constipation, asthenia (weakness and fatigue), diarrhea, abdominal pain, and dyspepsia (indigestion).

ZOFRAN (ANTINAUSEA)

Generic name: ondansetron.
Use: Zofran is used to prevent nausea and vomiting associated with cancer chemotherapy, radiation therapy, and surgery. The orally disintegrating tablets can be taken with or without water. Do not try to push the tablet through the foil backing. With dry hands, peel back the foil backing of one blister and gently remove the tablet. Immediately place a tablet on your tongue where it will dissolve in seconds and can be swallowed with saliva.
Possible side effects: If you experience any of the following serious side effects, stop taking Zofran and seek emergency medical attention: an allergic reaction (difficulty breathing; closing of the throat; swelling of the lips, tongue, or face; or hives), irregular heartbeat or chest pain, seizures or convulsions, or muscle cramps or uncontrollable movements.

Other less serious side effects may be more likely to occur. Continue to take Zofran and talk to your doctor if you experience headache, fatigue, drowsiness or dizziness, anxiety or agitation, or diarrhea or constipation.

INFORMATIVE DRUG RESOURCES

. . . . . .

Consumers Guide to Cancer Drugs, by Gail M. Wilkes, Terri B. Ades, and Irwin H. Krakoff (Jones & Bartlett, 2000).

This authoritative cancer drug guide from the American Cancer Society offers over 500 information-packed pages in a remarkably portable size; answers common drug-related questions in easy-to-understand language; and lists the most common drugs on the market today, giving the drug's action, how to take the drug, precautions, side effects, and other important facts.

The Essential Guide to Prescription Drugs, by James W. Long and James J. Rybacki (HarperCollins, 2002).

This valuable pharmaceutical reference provides information about dosages, side effects, precautions, treatment, interactions, and more, based on the latest FDA information.

PART IV

· ·

RESOURCES

· ·

National Breast Cancer Groups, Local Resources, Events, & Support Groups

. . . .

AMERICAN CANCER SOCIETY (ACS)

www.cancer.org

(800) ACS-2345 (Call the toll-free number for the location nearest you.)

The American Cancer Society is a national, community-based, voluntary health organization that works to eliminate cancer through prevention, life-saving treatment, and research, education, and direct service. Headquartered in Atlanta, Georgia, the ACS has state divisions and more than 3,400 local offices. Their 24-hour hotline provides prerecorded information on a range of topics.

Note: Website and hotline services available in Spanish.

Three useful patient-education and rehabilitation programs associated with the ACS include:

Cancer Survivors Network

www.acscsn.org

(877) 333-HOPE

Telephone and web-based services for cancer survivors, their families, caregivers, and friends. The telephone service provides survivors and families access to prerecorded discussions. The web-based section offers live online chat sessions, virtual support groups, prerecorded talk shows, and personal stories.

I Can Cope

A patient-education program that is designed to help patients, families, and friends cope with the day-to-day issues of living with cancer.

Look Good . . . Feel Better

www.lookgoodfeelbetter.org

This program was developed by the Cosmetic, Toiletry, and Fragrance Association Foundation in cooperation with the ACS and the National Cosmetology Association. It focuses on techniques that can help people undergoing cancer treatment improve their appearance.

Reach to Recovery

A rehabilitation program for women who have or have had breast cancer. The program helps breast cancer patients meet the physical, emotional, and cosmetic needs related to their disease and its treatment.

American Institute for Cancer Research (AICR)

www.aicr.org

1759 R Street NW

Washington, DC 20009

(800) 843-8114 or (202) 328-7744 in D.C.

The nation's third-largest cancer charity and a pioneer in the area of diet and nutrition as they relate to the prevention and treatment of cancer. The AICR has helped encourage innovative research related to diet, nutrition, and the prevention and treatment of cancer, while also serving as one of the country's leading sources for educational programs for cancer prevention. They provide information on diet, nutrition, and cancer. The AICR website includes the latest information and medical studies on cancer prevention and treatment. The AICR also publishes a quarterly newsletter and educational booklets on how people can help prevent cancer through proper nutrition.

The American Medical Association (AMA)

www.ama-assn.org

515 N. State Street

Chicago, IL 60610

(312) 464-5000

Founded more than 150 years ago, the AMA's work includes the development and promotion of standards in medical practice, research, and education; a strong advocacy agenda on behalf of patients and physicians; and the commitment to providing timely information on matters important to the health of America.

The AMA website has a detailed section for the general public, *AMA Health Insight*. Included in the section *Specific Conditions* is a detailed discussion about breast cancer and mammography. Learn the latest and most relevant news and information about AMA advocacy, initiatives, and events, as well as helpful tools, such as *Doctor Finder, Hospital Finder, Medical Group Practice Finder,* and *Medical Ethics.*

- *Hospital Select* is a hospital locator, providing information on virtually every hospital in the United States. This tool allows you to quickly and easily search for a hospital in your area.
- *AMA Physician Select* provides basic professional information on virtually every licensed physician in the United States and its possessions. Search for a physician by name or by medical specialty.
- *AMA Group Select* draws on the AMA's extensive database to help you find answers to your questions about the medical services in your community.

The Breast Cancer Fund (TBCF)
www.breastcancerfund.org
2107 O'Farrell Street
San Francisco, CA 94115
(415) 346-8223 or (800) 487-0492

The Breast Cancer Fund aims to end breast cancer through public education, advocacy, patient support initiatives, and research that promotes elimination of the preventable causes of the disease, including those in the environment; replacement of mammography with safer, more reliable screening methods; development of nontoxic treatments; and access to the best available medical care and information for everyone. TBCF sends out a monthly email alert to inform people of the latest breast cancer news and how you can take action to end the breast cancer epidemic. TBCF's website links to educational programs, where women can connect with critical information and ways to become more involved in the breast cancer issue.

Breast Cancer Resource Committee
http://afamerica.com/bcrc/
2005 Belmont Street NW
Washington, DC 20009
(202) 463-8015

Since its inception, BCRC has conducted more than 800 local and national breast cancer awareness programs targeting minority women and others who have little or no access to health care and treatment. The BCRC strives to:

- Provide comprehensive cancer awareness, education programs, and patient support targeting the African-American community (While its focus is the Washington, D.C., metropolitan area, it serves as a national resource, advocating mammography screening for African-American women aged 35 and older.)
- Promote and reinforce early detection and treatment of breast cancer through local, national, and international outreach
- Increase the participation of African-American women in early detection and screening for breast cancer
- Encourage major organizations to develop programs to educate all women about breast cancer

Cancer Care, Inc.
www.cancercare.org
275 Seventh Avenue
New York, NY 10001
(800) 813-HOPE (4673) or (212) 302-2400 in New York City

Cancer Care is a national, nonprofit agency that offers free support, information, financial assistance, and practical help to people with cancer and their loved ones. Services are provided by oncology social workers and are available in person, over the telephone, and through the agency's website. Cancer Care's reach also extends to professionals—providing education, information, and assistance. Cancer Care also offers on-site support groups, telephone conference and on-site education, and cancer care briefs.

Note: Sections of the website and some publications are available in Spanish. Staff can respond to calls and emails in Spanish.

Centers for Disease Control and Prevention (CDC)
http://www.cdc.gov/cancer/
CDC/DCPC
4770 Buford Highway, NE
MS K64
Atlanta, GA 30341
(888) 842-6355

The CDC provides the latest news on cancer research and information on federally funded cancer programs. For example, the National Breast and Cervical Cancer Detection program provides free or low-cost mammograms and Pap tests at several locations throughout the United States.

Note: Services available in Spanish.

Gilda's Club, Inc.
www.gildasclub.org
195 W. Houston Street
New York, NY 10014
(212) 647-9700

Gilda's Club, a free, nonprofit program, provides social and emotional support to cancer patients and their families and friends. Lectures, workshops, networking groups, special events, and a children's program are available. Twenty-five locations nationwide.

Note: Information available in Spanish.

National Action Plan on Breast Cancer
www.4woman.gov/napbc
Office on Women's Health
Department of Health and Human Services
Room 718F
200 Independence Avenue SW
Washington, DC 20201
(202) 401-9587

The NAPBC, coordinated by the Office on Women's Health, Department of Health and Human Services, coordinates efforts between government, nongovernmental agencies, groups, and individuals devoted to breast cancer in order to better educate and serve the breast cancer community.

It can provide you with links to information and educational resources on all breast cancer, advocacy groups, organizations, current research, and events.

Note: Information available in Spanish.

National Alliance of Breast Cancer Organizations (NABCO)

www.nabco.org

9 E. 37th Street, 10th Floor

New York, NY 10016

(888) 80-NABCO

To submit questions, send email to asknabco@aol.com. Time-sensitive questions requiring a personal reply should be sent to nabcoinfo@aol.com. NABCO is a nonprofit organization that provides information about breast cancer and acts as an advocate for the legislative concerns of breast cancer patients and survivors. NABCO maintains a list, organized by state, of phone numbers for support groups. NABCO provides assistance and referrals; it acts as a voice for the interests and concerns of breast cancer survivors and women at risk. It publishes a quarterly newsletter, *NABCO News,* and the annual Breast Cancer Resource List. NABCO also provides an email reminder service when it is time to schedule a breast exam.

The National Breast Cancer Foundation

www.nationalbreastcancer.org

One Hanover Park

16633 N. Dallas Parkway, Suite 600

Addison, TX 75001

The National Breast Cancer Foundation is a nonprofit charitable foundation whose primary purpose is to provide continuing public education on the early detection of breast cancer and free or low-cost mammography screenings to individuals and organizations, most particularly minority, low-income, homeless, and working poor women. The NBCF website provides recent news articles as well as basic information on breast cancer.

National Cancer Institute

http://cis.nci.nih.gov/ (note: no "www" needed)

(800) 4-CANCER

The National Cancer Institute coordinates the National Cancer Program, which conducts and supports research, training, health information dissemination, and other programs with respect to the cause, diagnosis, prevention, and treatment of cancer, rehabilitation from cancer, and the continuing care of cancer patients and the families of cancer patients.

Note: Website and hotline services available in Spanish; deaf and hearing-impaired phone services; publication catalogue lists materials in English and Spanish, and with low reading levels designed for patients, their families, health care providers, and the general public.

NCI Cancer Information Service (CIS)
(800) 4-CANCER

Call Mon.–Fri., 9 A.M.–5 P.M., EST to speak with a live person; recorded information about cancer is available 24 hours per day.

The CIS, a public hotline to interpret and explain cancer research findings in clear and understandable language, serves the public through two programs: a toll-free telephone service and an outreach program. Through its toll-free phone service, the CIS provides accurate, up-to-date information on cancer to patients and their families, health professionals, and the general public. The CIS outreach program serves as a resource to communities and organizations by providing technical assistance and materials to support cancer education activities.

CancerNet
http://cancernet.nci.nih.gov/ (no "www" needed)

CancerNet provides comprehensive information for anyone with a question about cancer, for particular patients, caregivers, health care professionals, researchers, and others. The breast cancer section of CancerNet (http://cancernet.nci.nih.gov/cancer_types/breast_cancer.shtml) provides detailed information on breast cancer statistics, risk factors, diagnosis, treatment, coping with side effects of treatment, support groups, and so on.

Note: Services available in Spanish: http://cancernet.nci.nih.gov/sp_menu.htm (no "www" needed).

National Comprehensive Cancer Network (NCCN)
www.nccn.org
50 Huntingdon Pike, Suite 200
Rockledge, PA 19046
(215) 728-4788
(888) 909-NCCN (patient information service)

The NCCN is a nonprofit corporation that was established in 1995 to enhance the leadership role of member institutions in the managed health care environment. The NCCN seeks to support and strengthen the mission of member institutions in three basic areas: to provide state-of-the-art cancer care to the greatest number of patients in need; to advance the state of the art in cancer prevention, screening, diagnosis, and treatment through excellence in basic and clinical research; and to enhance the effectiveness and efficiency of cancer care delivery through the ongoing collection, synthesis, and analysis of outcomes data. The NCCN and the American Cancer Society have partnered to translate the *NCCN Practice Guidelines in Oncology* into a patient-friendly resource outlining appropriate treatment.

National Institutes of Health (NIH)
www.nih.gov
National Institutes of Health
Bethesda, MD 20892
(301) 496-4000

A component of the U.S. Department of Health and Human Services. It consists of 25 institutes and centers that conduct medical research for the federal government. Services include health information, news and events, and scientific resources.

Note: Information available in Spanish.

The Susan G. Komen Breast Cancer Foundation
www.komen.org, www.breastcancerinfo.com,
and www.racceforthecure.com
5005 LBJ Freeway, Suite 370
Dallas, TX 75244
(972) 855-1600 or (800) I'M AWARE, Mon.–Fri., 9 A.M.–4:30 P.M., CST

The Susan G. Komen Breast Cancer Foundation's mission is to eradicate breast cancer as a life-threatening disease by advancing research, education, screening, and treatment. This organization operates a national toll-free breast cancer helpline that is answered by trained volunteers whose lives have been personally touched by breast cancer. Breast health and breast cancer materials, including pamphlets, brochures, booklets, posters, videos, CD-ROMs, fact sheets, and community outreach materials are available. Information on the Komen Race for the Cure series is also available.

Note: Staff can respond to calls in Spanish, and some publications are available in Spanish.

The Wellness Community

www.wellness-community.org

35 E. Seventh Street, Suite 412

Cincinnati, OH 45202

(888) 793-WELL

The Wellness Community consists of more than 20 centers nationwide, providing emotional support, education, and hope for people with cancer. The Wellness Community provides a full range of support services to cancer patients and their families in a comfortable, homelike setting, completely free of charge. They offer drop-in and ongoing support groups, networking groups for specific types of cancer, educational workshops, stress management sessions, a weekly online support group, online chat groups, lectures by experts in the field of oncology, and social gatherings.

Women's Information Network Against Breast Cancer (WINABC)

www.winabc.org/newweb/index.htm

536 S. Second Avenue, Suite K

Covina, CA 91723-3043

(626) 332-2255

The goal of the WINABC, a national nonprofit organization founded by Betsy Mullen, is to increase public awareness about breast cancer and ensure that individuals from all socioeconomic backgrounds have rapid access to state-of-the-art education, support, and information about this disease.

WINABC provides up-to-date information on breast cancer diagnosis, treatment, and recovery as well as a comprehensive list of free services offered to breast cancer patients and their families. Trained survivors offer information and peer support via a national hotline.

Note: Hotline services available in Spanish and Filipino.

Y-ME National Breast Cancer Organization

www.y-me.org

212 W. Van Buren Street, 5th Floor

Chicago, IL 60607

(800) 221-2141, available 24 hours a day

Y-ME's aim is to increase breast cancer awareness and ensure that no one faces breast cancer alone by providing information, empowerment, and peer support. Y-ME serves women with breast cancer and their families through their national hotline, open-door groups, early detection workshops, and support programs. Y-ME also offers a matching service that can bring a newly diagnosed breast cancer patient together with a survivor with a similar diagnostic or pathologic profile to facilitate understanding of the treatment process and to provide support. Numerous local chapter offices are located throughout the United States.

Note: A section of the website, a toll-free hotline, and publications are available in Spanish.

PATIENT EMPOWERMENT
RESOURCES & INFORMATION
. . . .

The following resource list is a compilation of educational pamphlets, websites, books, magazines, newsletters, and hotlines. The list is divided into categories in order to make finding information easier. It is by no means an exhaustive list of available resources for women with breast cancer but is intended to be a valuable starting point for women wishing to make informed and active decisions regarding their medical care. Many of the following resources offer services, website access, and printed material at no cost.

Free resources are indicated by the □ *icon.*

GENERAL BREAST CANCER RESOURCES

□ **The Association of Cancer Online Resources (ACOR)**
www.acor.org
173 Duane Street, Suite 3A
New York, NY 10013-3334
(212) 226-5525
The acor.org cancer information system currently offers access to more than 140 electronic mailing lists and a wide variety of websites. The mail-

ing lists are specifically designed to be public online support groups, providing information and community to tens of thousands of patients, caregivers, or anyone looking for answers about cancer and related disorders.

□ **AMC Cancer Research Center's Cancer Information Line**
1600 Pierce Street
Denver, CO 90214
(800) 525-3777, Mon.–Fri., 8:30 A.M.–5:00 P.M., MST

Professional cancer counselors provide answers to questions about cancer and give compassionate support and advice. They will also mail free publications on request.

Note: Equipped for deaf and hearing-impaired callers.

Breast Cancer? Breast Health! The Wise Woman Way **(Wise Woman Herbal Series, book 4), by Susun S. Weed and Christine Northrup, M.D.** (Ash Tree, 1997).

This book should be required reading for all women—whether or not you have cancer. The smart-as-a-whip herbalist Susun Weed provides positive and well-researched suggestions for living a healthy lifestyle. Her suggestions have helped many women withstand the effects of chemotherapy and strengthen their immune system to help their bodies fight cancer (with appropriate warnings and toxicities mentioned in the few cases where appropriate).

□ **The Breast Cancer Decision Guide**
www.bcdg.org

This website was developed by the U.S. Department of Defense for both military and civilian families. The site gives general breast cancer information, guidelines for breast cancer screening, and explanations of different types of therapies, including surgery and complementary surgeries. Users answer a series of medical and nonmedical questions and receive case-specific information on treatment options, survival rates, recurrences, and so on. Users may need to refer to mammogram, biopsy, or other breast-imaging results to answer some questions.

Breast Cancer: What You Should Know (But May Not Be Told) about Prevention, Diagnosis, and Treatment, **by Steve Austin and Cathy Hitchcock** (Prima, 1994).

For women who want to actively participate in their diagnosis and treatment, this book explores pertinent medical information about breast cancer by both conventional and alternative medicine. The beautiful illustrations and charts are especially helpful.

☐ **Breastdoc.com**
www.breastdoc.com
The website of Dr. Deborah Axelrod (friend of Rosie O'Donnell's and chief of St. Vincent's Comprehensive Breast Center). Features up-to-the-minute information on new techniques in the diagnosis and treatment of breast cancer, as well as updates on risk reduction and lecture and event information. My favorite feature is "Pen Pal Buddies," a support system pairing newly diagnosed women with women who've experienced similar treatments.

☐ **Cancerandcareers.org**
www.cancerandcareers.org
(212) 685-5955, ext. 15
This must-see website for coworkers and employers of women with breast cancer was created by the Cosmetic Executive Women (a nonprofit organization representing women in the U.S. and European beauty industries). Work doesn't stop once you've been diagnosed with cancer, and over 80 percent of cancer survivors return to work after treatment. This sleek website gives employers and coworkers the tools—articles, news, charts, checklists, tips, and a community of experts, patients, and survivors—to help women continue to work through treatment.

The Cancer Dictionary, by Roberta Altman and Michael J. Sarg, M.D. (textbook) (Facts on File, 1999, $55).
Altman, a former cancer patient, and Sarg, an oncologist at St. Vincent's Hospital in New York, provide an extensive resource for cancer patients, their families, and people interested in prevention.

☐ **CancerFax**
(800) 624-2511 or (301) 402-5874, follow the voice-prompt instructions
This fax-on-demand service allows access to NCI's Physician's Data Query system via fax machine, 24 hours a day, 7 days a week, at no charge other than the charge for the fax call. Two versions of the treatment infor-

mation are available: one for health care professionals and the other for patients, family, or the general public. To obtain instructions and the list of necessary codes, call (301) 402-5874. If there are problems with the fax, call (800) 624-7890 or obtain code information by phone through the Cancer Information Service, (800) 4-CANCER, or on the web at http://cancernet.nci.nih.gov/.

Note: Material available in Spanish.

Diagnosis Guide: Your Guide through the First Few Months, by Wendy Schlessel Harpham, M.D. (Norton, 1997).

This book is for anyone who has just received a cancer diagnosis (not specific to breast cancer), as well as for those who care about them. It covers everything that you need to digest during those first few months, in an easy-to-understand, straightforward manner. It is written with medical expertise and geared toward the woman with no prior knowledge of cancer.

Dr. Susan Love's Breast Book, by Susan Love, M.D., with Karen Lindsey (Perseus Book Group, revised 2000). Available through SusanLoveMD. com, PO Box 846, Pacific Palisades, CA 90272, (310) 230-1712.

Dr. Susan Love's Breast Book, like the first two editions, pulls no punches. It's packed with the latest information on breast cancer diagnosis, treatment, and research and is recommended for anyone who has been diagnosed with breast cancer and wants a clear explanation of the whole picture. This book is the "bible" for breast health and extremely helpful for the newly diagnosed woman. SusanLoveMD.com is an up-to-the-minute website devoted to original, in-depth, health-related information and women's midlife health concerns, including breast cancer and menopause.

□ **The Feminist Majority Foundation's Breast Cancer Home Page (FMF)**
www.feminist.org/other/bc/bchome.html
The FMF's breast cancer page reviews dozens of breast cancer sites, offers the latest feminist news on breast cancer and info on who to call when you're diagnosed with breast cancer, on clinical trials, and on how to find and participate in a local walk or road race. FMF, which was founded in 1987, is a cutting-edge organization dedicated to women's equality, reproductive health, and nonviolence.

☐ *For Single Women with Breast Cancer* (1994). Call (800) 221-2141.

Y-ME pamphlet offers practical guidance and emotional support for women without partners or those who live alone.

☐ **The National Consortium of Breast Centers**
http://breastcare.org
PO Box 1334
Warsaw, IN 46581-1334
(219) 267-8058

This website provides information on locating breast centers and other facilities involved in breast health care. Patients may search a database of breast health facilities by city or state. The website also helps users locate services to enhance the administration, operation, and marketing of breast health facilities.

☐ **National Women's Health Information Center (NWHIC)**
www.4women.gov
(800) 994-WOMAN, Mon.–Fri., 9 A.M.–6 P.M., EST

This website is sponsored by the Office on Women's Health in the Department of Health and Human Services. It provides a broad array of reliable, commercial-free health publications and referrals to health-related organizations for women.

Note: Some of this information is available in Spanish and equipped for deaf and hearing-impaired callers.

☐ **PDQ (Physician Data Query)**
http://cancernet.nci.nih.gov (no "www" is necessary)
(800) 4-CANCER

The computerized cancer database of the National Cancer Institute provides information on treatment, organizations, and doctors involved in cancer care and a listing of more than 1,500 clinical trials that are open to patient accrual. The database is accessible by a computer equipped with a modem or by fax.

☐ **University of Pennsylvania's OncoLink**
http://oncolink.upenn.edu/
University of Pennsylvania Cancer Center
3400 Spruce Street, 2 Donner
Philadelphia, PA 19104-4283

Maintained by the University of Pennsylvania Cancer Center, Onco-Link is full of well-referenced, carefully approved information on cancer treatment and survivorship. The site also offers general information, discussion of medical supportive care, issues related to the treatment of cancer, and information on various genetic research studies. This site gets rave reviews for its breast cancer content but is an excellent resource for any cancer patient.

Note: Worldwide resources available.

☐ *What You Need to Know About Breast Cancer* (98-1556, August 1998). Call (800) 4-CANCER.

The NCIs most comprehensive pamphlet on breast cancer (44 pages), *What You Need to Know About Breast Cancer* covers symptoms, diagnosis, treatment, emotional issues, questions to ask your doctor, and a glossary of terms.

☐ **Women's Cancer Resource Center**
www.wcrc.org
5741 Telegraph Avenue
Oakland, CA 94609
(510) 420-7900 or (888) 421-7900

I admit, I'm biased about the services that WCRC provides because I volunteer there. Many of the services are Bay Area–focused, but services such as the peer referral network, legal services, and resource library help women nationwide and around the world. Here's a brief look at WCRC's services:

- *Educational forums and workshops:* Forums and workshop topics are offered on a range of topics. Past workshop topics include mainstream and alternative treatment options, breast implants, yoga, qigong, stress reduction, and community education on the link between cancer and the environment.
- *Free therapy program:* In 1995, the Center initiated a free therapy program for low-income women with cancer. This service provides up to 6 months of free weekly psychotherapy sessions with licensed women therapists.
- *Information and referral hotline:* Several hundred calls from women with cancer, their friends, family, and loved ones come in to the hotline each month; 35 percent of them are from outside of California. Vol-

unteers who staff the lines provide information on local support groups and services, treatment options, and information on local physicians and other health care providers.

- *In-home support services:* The Betts program is the only program of its kind in the San Francisco Bay Area. Linking volunteers with low-income women in the community seeking practical and emotional support, this program provides crucial support to women with cancer.
- *Legal services:* Periodically, WCRC presents legal workshops, which assist in understanding current issues facing women's health.
- *Peer referral network:* Through our peer referral network, callers are linked to women with similar medical diagnoses, ethnic background, language, sexual orientation, and treatment choices. By connecting women with peers who have "been there," this service provides invaluable information and emotional support to over 1,500 callers each year.
- *Peer support groups:* The Center offers a number of peer-based support groups. Trained facilitators with experience run our groups.
- *Resource library:* WCRC's comprehensive lending library provides accessible, up-to-date information on cancer treatment and women's health issues. The library includes more than 3,000 volumes, clipping files, periodicals, pamphlets, audio and videocassettes, and medical database and Internet access. The library is one of the few that offers materials for women whose first language is other than English, and information on the full spectrum of both mainstream and complementary therapies. Supervised library volunteers research and produce several hundred information packets each year for women who are homebound, live out of the area, or are unable to utilize the library in person.

Note: Hotline and resources are available in Spanish; equipped for deaf and hearing-impaired callers; lesbian support services.

BONE MARROW TRANSPLANT

☐ **American Bone Marrow Donor Registry (ABMDR)**
www.abmdr.org
(800) 726-2824
ABMDR coordinates and processes patient-search requests, provides comprehensive assistance to patients and physicians throughout the search

process, and helps to minimize the costs associated with donor recruitment and the patient-search process. Two registries of volunteer bone marrow donors exist to help patients seeking a transplant. Your transplant center can help you find a donor utilizing these registries.

Bone and Marrow Transplant Information Network (BMT)
www.bmtinfonet.org
2900 Skokie Valley Road, Suite B
Highland Park, IL 60035
(888) 597-7674 or (847) 433-3313, during regular business hours
BMT's team of more than 200 bone marrow transplant survivors provides emotional support before, during and after the transplant process. The website also offers a drug database, news bulletin, resource directory, guide to transplant centers, and links to help solve insurance difficulties. *Bone Marrow Transplant—A Book of Basics for Patients,* by Susan K. Stewart, and paper copies of BMT's newsletter are also available.

☐ **National Marrow Donor Program**
www.marrow.org
3001 Broadway Street NE, Suite 500
Minneapolis, MN 55413-1753
(800) 526-7809
The National Marrow Donor Program (NMDP) is an international leader in the facilitation of unrelated marrow and blood stem cell transplantation. It is the only organization that offers a single point of access for all sources of stem cells used in transplantation: marrow, peripheral blood, and umbilical cord blood. At any given time, the NMDP offers hope to more than 3,000 patients searching its registry.

Note: Resources available in Spanish, Korean, Chinese, Japanese, and Vietnamese.

COMPLEMENTARY/ALTERNATIVE MEDICINE (CAM)

The Alternative Medicine Handbook: The Complete Reference Guide to Alternative and Complementary Therapies, by Barrie R. Cassileth (Norton, 1999).

The book is written for those without a Ph.D. or M.D. following their name, which translates to information that is extremely easy to understand. Provides a comprehensive evaluation of the science behind several alternative and holistic approaches that can help patients get through physically and psychologically difficult medical treatment such as breast cancer treatment.

☐ **Amazon: Alternative Therapies for Breast Cancer**
To join, send an email message to: listserv@listserv.aol.com.
In the body of the message type: Subscribe Amazon [Your Name]
List owners: Bonnie Bedford at Bedford@islandnet.com and Michelle Lowe at mishlowe37@aol.com

The Amazon list is for women who are using alternative treatments as the primary treatment for breast cancer. This is a supportive forum for women to discuss any aspect of the disease (physical, mental, or spiritual), body image, treatments they are trying, and treatments they are interested in learning about.

☐ **The Annie Appleseed Project**
www.annieappleseedproject.org
Acts to spread news, views and information about access to alternative and complementary cancer therapies. Many contributors to the reports listed on the site are patients.
Note: African-American-specific studies, articles, and other information available.

☐ **Cancer Control Society (CCS)**
www.cancercontrolsociety.com
2043 N. Berendo Street
Los Angeles, CA 90027
(323) 663-7801
Since 1973, the CCS has brought information to thousands of patients and their families. Every Labor Day weekend, CCS sponsors the Cancer Control Convention, featuring doctors and other experts in alternative medicine sharing their latest findings for treating cancer and other degenerative diseases. Throughout the year, the CCS distributes books, videos, and tapes on everything in alternative medicine from amygdalin to zinc. CCS also publishes its *Green Sheet,* a directory of doctors practicing alternative medicine, and its *Patient Sheet,* a list of names, addresses, and phone

numbers of patients who claim their cancer was controlled by alternative therapies.

□ **Charlotte Maxwell Complementary Clinic (CMCC)**
www.charlottemaxwell.org
5691 Telegraph Avenue
Oakland, CA 94609
(510) 601-6315

A Bay Area clinic for low-income women with cancer, dedicated to the concept that all women deserve access to basic medical care, support services, and complementary therapies such as acupuncture, Chinese herbs, massage, and homeopathy. CMCC also offers social work assistance, transportation to and from clinic appointments, fresh organic produce and bread, and educational workshops. The In-Home Comfort Care Program provides complementary alternative medicine (CAM) treatments for those clients with end-stage cancer who are too weak to come to the Clinic. The Post-Treatment Program extends CAM treatments, emotional support, and educational workshops to women living with cancer who have finished their allopathic treatment and have no signs of recurrence. The Carol Zambel Treatment Access Fund is available for women who require financial assistance in obtaining additional CAM treatments, herbs, and medication not currently offered by CMCC.

Note: Multilingual social worker available.

Choices in Healing: Integrating the Best of Conventional and Complementary Approaches to Cancer, by **Michael Lerner** (MIT Press, 1996).

Lerner investigates the extent to which various cancer therapies work, mostly by reviewing so-called serious research and examining cancer treatments from different angles. In areas where scientific studies contradict each other, he doesn't draw unsubstantiated conclusions. He manages to give specific guidelines for dealing with cancer without advocating any one therapy too much. The tone of the book is honest, warm, caring, and personal without being overly sentimental. Best of all, it inspires hope.

□ **The National Center for Complementary and Alternative Medicine (NCAAM)**
http://nccam.nih.gov
PO Box 7923

Gaithersburg, MD 20898

(888) 644-6226

Contact the NCCAM for the *Considering Complementary and Alternative Medicine?* fact sheet, which provides helpful hints and questions to consider when choosing an alternative health care practitioner. The NCCAM also facilitates and supports basic and applied research of complementary and alternative medicine (CAM) modalities. It sponsors training for researchers and publishes information about CAM therapies for practitioners and the public.

□ **Institute for Health and Healing Resource Center**

www.cpmc.org/services/ihh/services/resource

California Pacific Medical Center

San Francisco, CA 94120

(415) 600-3681

The Health and Healing Resource Center (A Planetree Affiliate Library) offers a wealth of resources to assist you in making informed health care decisions. They offer the Healing Store, with vitamins, herbs, natural body care products, books, and other carefully selected items. The library also provides, for a fee, computer-searched information packets on any health topic by mail.

□ **Swallows-L**

To join, send an email message to: listserv@techunix.technion.ac.il

In the body of the message type: subscribe SWALLOWS-L

[Your Name]

List owner: Belinda Berry, berry@flyingcameraco.demon.co.uk

www.flyingcameraco.demon.co.uk/Swallows.htm

This online discussion list was formed for the benefit of those who wish to use conventional and alternative therapies for breast cancer in an integrated, complementary manner.

Third Opinion: An International Directory to Alternate Therapy Centers for the Treatment and Prevention of Cancer and Other Degenerative Diseases, by **John M. Fink** (Avery, 1997).

An international directory to alternative therapy centers for the treatment and prevention of cancer and other degenerative diseases.

DIET AND NUTRITION

☐ **Cancer Research Foundation of America**
www.preventcancer.org
1600 Duke Street, Suite 110
Alexandria, VA 22314
1-800-227-CRFA
(703) 836-4412

The Cancer Research Foundation of America seeks to prevent cancer by funding research and providing educational materials on early detection and nutrition.

The Cancer Survival Cookbook, **by Donna Weihofen and Christina Marino** (Wiley, 1997). Available in bookstores or call (800) 848-2793.

This book is packed with nourishing, easy-to-prepare recipes, as well as invaluable advice on overcoming eating problems that often accompany cancer treatment.

☐ *Eating Hints for Cancer Patients* (98-2079, 1998). Go to http://cancernet.nci.nih.gov/eating_hints/eatintro.html or call (800) 4-CANCER.

The National Cancer Institute has prepared this collection of suggestions and recipes to help you learn more about your diet needs and how to manage eating problems. This guide is mainly for patients who are still receiving cancer treatment. However, it also may be useful after you finish treatment. Refer to it any time you find that eating well is a challenge.

A Guide to Good Nutrition During and After Chemotherapy and Radiation, **by Saundra N. Aker and Polly Lennsen** (1998). Available from the Fred Hutchinson Cancer Research Center Clinical Nutrition Program, 1124 Columbia Street, Room E211, Seattle, WA 98104, (206) 667-4834.

This guide offers a practical approach to nutrition.

EARLY DETECTION, MAMMOGRAMS, AND IMAGING PROCEDURES

The American Breast Cancer Foundation (ABCF)
www.abcf.org
1055 Taylor Avenue, Suite 201A
Baltimore, MD 21286
(877) 539-2543

It is ABCF's mission to ensure access to preventative and diagnostic measures concerning breast cancer to all women, no matter their age, race, or financial challenges. This includes access to breast cancer screening services, the ever-important search for a cure, and support services for breast cancer patients and their families after diagnosis.

☐ *Digital Mammography* (NABCO, January 2001). Go to www.nabco. org or call (800) 80-NABCO.

This fact sheet explains digital mammography and offers updated information on its potential.

☐ *Things to Know About Quality Mammograms* (AHCPR Publication No. 95-0634, October 1994). Available from Agency for Health Care Policy and Research, Publications Clearinghouse, PO Box 8547, Silver Spring, MD 20907, (800) 358-9295.

Still current, this consumer pamphlet details the U.S. government's Agency for Health Care Policy and Research recommendations for getting the best mammogram.

Note: Available in Spanish.

☐ **Food and Drug Administration (FDA)**
Listing of Certified Mammography Facilities
http://www.fda.gov/cdrh/mammography/certified.html
(800) 4-CANCER

Call the NCI for the nearest FDA-certified mammography provider or to check the status of your imaging center. The list of FDA Certified Mammography Facilities is updated weekly.

☐ **Radiology Info**

www.radiologyinfo.org

The public information website of the Radiological Society of North America (RSNA) and the American College of Radiology (ACR). Provides information on mammography and other imaging exams such as ultrasound and MRI. The mammogram section (www.radiologyinfo.org/content/mammogram.htm) includes information on common uses of a mammogram, how to prepare for a mammogram, how the exam is performed, and benefits and risks of having a mammogram. All sections are written clearly, and many contain photographs.

GENETIC TESTING

Breakthrough: The Race to Find the Breast Cancer Gene, by Kevin Davies and Michael White (Wiley, 1996).

Kevin Davies, the editor of the journal *Nature Genetics,* and Michael White, a science journalist, have chronicled the search for BRCA1, the gene for "heritable" breast cancer, in an enlightening book.

☐ **FORCE (Facing Our Risk of Cancer Empowered)**

www.facingourrisk.org

934 N. University Drive, PMB No. 213

Coral Springs, FL 33071

A nonprofit organization for women whose family history and genetic status put them at high risk of getting ovarian and/or breast cancer, and for members of families in which this risk is present. The website provides information and suggests links on topics related to breast cancer risk, diagnosis, treatment, coping with the loss of a loved one, and more.

☐ **InTouchlive.com**

www.intouchlive.com

This website, from the same people who publish *InTouch* magazine, provides both clinical and basic information on cancer, heredity, and the roles genes play in the development of various cancers, on their Genetics of Cancer page. (Click on "Cancer Genetics.")

☐ *Genetic Testing for Cancer Risk: Its Your Choice* (Sponsored by the National Action Plan on Breast Cancer). Call (800) 4-CANCER.

Hosted by Cokie Roberts, this 14-minute video gives an overview of the risks and benefits of being tested for genetic susceptibility to breast and ovarian cancer.

Note: Companion brochure available.

GROUP-SPECIFIC RESOURCES

African American

☐ **African American Breast Cancer Alliance (AABCA)**
www.geocities.com/aabcainc
PO Box 8981
Minneapolis, MN 55408
(612) 644-1224
AABCA's website includes regional and national networks, support and advocacy for black women with breast cancer and their families, information and referrals, education, and a newsletter.

African American Women in Touch
(219) 284-6944
Empowers the female African-American community to take a more active role in meeting their health needs.

BlackWomensHealth.com
www.blackwomenshealth.com
The website's home page offers news and highlights on selected health and wellness issues, as well as links to information on specific health topics, nutrition and fitness, spiritual and mental health, and personal finance issues. The breast cancer page includes an overview of the disease with statistics, risk factors, detailed descriptions of mammography, breast self-exams and clinical breast examinations, a discussion of different forms of biopsies and breast cancer treatments, and contact details for support and information.

The Black Women's Health Book: Speaking for Ourselves, **edited by Evelyn C. White** (Seal Press, 1994).

More than 50 black women write about the health issues (not breast cancer–specific) that affect them and their communities. An empowering book for any woman wanting to take charge of her health and treatment.

Breast Cancer Resource Committee
http://afamerica.com/bcrc/
2005 Belmont Street NW
Washington, DC 20009
(202) 463-8015

Since its inception, BCRC has conducted more than 800 local and national breast cancer awareness programs targeting minority women and others who have little or no access to health care and treatment. Recognizing the dire need among African-American women to find solace and support from other African-American women diagnosed with and/or treated for breast cancer, BCRC established Rise-Sister-Rise, a 16-week comprehensive program conducted by faculty who are trained professionals in the psychological healing aspects of breast cancer. This Afrocentric women's group embraces the principles of African spirituality and provides a loving, nurturing, and supportive environment where African-American women can receive counseling and support for breast cancer diagnosis.

☐ **The Celebrating Life Foundation**
www.celebratinglife.org
PO Box 224076
Dallas, TX 75222-4076
(800) 207-0992

The Celebrating Life Foundation has initiated and participated in seminars, workshops, forums, health fairs, and other programs and activities related to breast cancer awareness and education both locally and nationally.

Celebrating Life: African American Women Speak Out About Breast Cancer, by Sylvia Dunnavant (Usfi, 1995). Can be found used on www.amazon.com.

Dunnavant poignantly relates encouraging survivors' personal stories (mostly in the survivors' own words), allowing the reader to feel the pains, the fears, and the joys expressed. The book is about survivors "celebrating life," and that celebration of life is reflected in all of the beautiful photographs.

Men In Action Against Breast Cancer
Breast Cancer Resource Committee
http://afamerica.com/bcrc/
2005 Belmont Street NW
Washington, DC 20009
(202) 463-8015

Organized in 1996 by BCRC, "Men in Action" harnesses the enormous, and often untapped, support resource that exists in the African-American community—its men. Since its inception, "Men in Action" has developed outreach and education programs to inform African-American women and men about the risk of breast cancer in their community. Incorporating unique activities and traditional "meeting grounds" for men, for example, athletics, music, and so on, BCRC has helped to create new opportunities to spread the breast cancer message.

☐ National Black Women's Health Project
www.nbwhp.org
600 Pennsylvania Avenue SE, Suite 310
Washington, DC 20003
(202) 543-9311

A national grassroots advocacy organization with local chapters and self-help groups.

☐ Sisters Network
www.sistersnetworkinc.org
8787 Woodway Drive, Suite 4206
Houston, TX 77063
(713) 781-0255

Sisters Network is the first nationwide African-American breast cancer survivors group committed to increasing local and national attention to the devastating impact that breast cancer has on the African-American community.

Asian

Asian Health Services (AHS)

www.ahschc.org/defaultothers.htm
818 Webster Street
Oakland, CA 94607
(510) 986-6830

A nationally recognized comprehensive primary care community health center and pioneer in establishing models of health care service and advocacy for the Asian and Pacific Islander community.

National Asian Women's Health Organization (NAWHO)

www.nawho.org
250 Montgomery Street, Suite 900
San Francisco, CA 94104
(415) 989-9747

NAWHO is working to improve the health status of Asian women and families through research, education, leadership, and public policy programs. Publications on subjects such as reproductive rights, breast and cervical cancer, and tobacco control are available.

Note: Resources available in English, Cantonese, Laotian, Vietnamese, and Korean.

Vietnamese Community Health Promotion Project

http://medicine.ucsf.edu/vchpp
44 Page Street, Suite 500
San Francisco, CA 94102
(415) 476-0557

Vietnamese Community Health Promotion Project wants to improve the health of Vietnamese living in the United States by advocating for change in government policies.

Note: Resources available in Vietnamese and English.

Disabled Women

☐ **Breast Health Access for Women with Disabilities (BHAWD)**
www.bhawd.org

c/o Alta Bates Summit Medical Center
Herrick Campus/Rehabilitation Services
2001 Dwight Way, 2nd Floor
Berkeley, CA 94704
(510) 204-4866

BHAWD was founded in 1995 in response to the lack of access to breast health care for women with disabilities. At the BHAWD clinic, women with disabilities, 20 years and older, are given free clinical breast exams, self breast exam education and training, and referral for a mammogram, if appropriate.

Note: Equipped for deaf and hearing-impaired callers.

Families and Children

□ *A Shared Purpose: A Guide for Daughters Whose Mothers Have Advanced Breast Cancer* (Cancer Care, 1998). Go to www.cancercare.org or call (800) 813-HOPE.

This 18-page pamphlet answers questions about advanced breast cancer and addresses feelings and emotions that mothers and daughters may face.

□ **Caringkids**

To subscribe, go to http://oncolink.upenn.edu/psychosocial/

An online support group for children with an ill person in their life. It offers a monitored, open forum where kids may exchange information, share their feelings, and make friends with other kids dealing with similar issues.

□ **Helping Children Cope Program**

www.cancercare.org
(800) 813-HOPE

Offers support groups and telephone counseling for children with a parent who has cancer. Also available is *Helping Children Cope When a Parent Has Cancer,* a 12-page pamphlet to help your children.

□ *Kemoshark,* by H. Elizabeth King, illustrated by Diane Willford Steele (1995). Available from www.kidscope.org or KIDSCOPE, 3400 Peachtree Road, Suite 703, Atlanta, GA 30326, (404) 253-0001.

A colorfully illustrated, 14-page pamphlet to help children understand chemotherapy when a parent is undergoing treatment.

☐ **Kids Count Too**
www.cancer.org
(800) ACS-2345 (for the program nearest you)
The American Cancer Society runs a 6-session program for children age 3 through teens coping with a parent's cancer.

☐ **Kids Konnected**
www.kidskonnected.org
(800) 462-9273
Susan G. Komen Foundation runs *Kids Konnected,* a support group for children whose mothers have breast cancer. Call for locations.

☐ *Kids Talk—Kids Speak Out About Breast Cancer,* by Laura Numeroff and Wendy S. Harpham (Samsung Telecommunications America and Sprint PCS, 1998). Call (800) IM-AWARE.
Clever short stories told by children about living with a mother with breast cancer, for children aged 10 and younger.

☐ **Mothers Supporting Daughters with Breast Cancer**
www.mothersdaughters.org
21710 Bayshore Road
Chestertown, MD 21620-4401
(410) 778-1982
MSDBC is a national nonprofit organization cofounded by a mother and her daughter. The support services provided by this organization are designed to help mothers who have daughters battling breast cancer. Also available is *Handbook for Mothers Supporting Daughters with Breast Cancer* (1995), a 26-page handbook that gives practical advice and sources of information to the mothers of women with breast cancer.

The Paper Chain, by Claire Blake, Eliza Blanchard, and Kathy Parkinson (Health Press, 1998). Available at bookstores or call (800) 643-BOOK.
For children ages 3 to 8, this book relays the emotions of two young boys whose mom has breast cancer. The short story includes the mother going to the hospital, having less energy for her sons, and their changed lifestyle. The book encourages hope and warm feelings.

☐ *Taking Time: Support for People with Cancer and the People Who Care About Them.* Call (800) 4-CANCER.

A free National Cancer Institute pamphlet addressing the concerns of caring for people with cancer.

□ *Talking about Your Cancer: A Parents Guide to Helping Children Cope.* Call (800) FOX-CHASE.

An 18-minute videotape from the Fox Chase Cancer Center that helps parents with cancer explain their diagnosis to their children, offering reassurance to families struggling with a new diagnosis and information for those already coping with cancer.

□ *When the Woman You Love Has Breast Cancer* (Y-ME, 1994). Available through www.y-me.org or call (800) 221-2141.

A Y-ME pamphlet that helps partners give emotional support to their loved ones.

Jewish

American Jewish Congress

www.ajcongress.org/pages/w_health.htm

Offers press releases focusing on Jewish women and the genetics of breast cancer. *Understanding Genetics of Breast Cancer for Jewish Women* (1997) was compiled as a follow-up to the First Leadership Conference on Jewish Women's Health Issues, to answer questions about the hereditary risk of breast cancer.

Latina

Breastlink.com, Integrated Breast Cancer Care

www.breastlink.com

Information on a variety of topics related to diagnosis and treatment of breast cancer, including a link for Latinas.

Note: Resources available in Spanish.

Cancer Links

www.cancerlinks.com

Links to Spanish breast cancer information, including an excellent section on inflammatory breast cancer.

Note: Resources available in Spanish.

COSSMHO
www.cossmho.org
1501 Sixteenth Street NW
Washington, DC 20036
(202) 387-5000

A national coalition of Hispanic health and human service organizations. Also conducts its own research on Latinas' experience with cancer services.
Note: Resources available in Spanish.

Margaret Cruz Latina Breast Cancer Foundation
www.mcruzlbcf.com
7 Joost Avenue, Suite 101
San Francisco, CA 94131
(415) 239-4802

This foundation's mission is to facilitate access to education, health care, and emotional support for Latinas who have been diagnosed with cancer. Although psycho/social services and much of the patient education services target women living in the Bay Area, books, pamphlets, a resource guide, and a website are available for women living anywhere.
Note: Resources available in Spanish.

The National Alliance for Hispanic Health
www.hispanichealth.org
1501 Sixteenth Street NW
Washington, DC 20036
(866) 783-2645 or (202) 387-5000

Comprehensive general health resource for Hispanics, including health fact sheets, toll-free helplines, publications for consumers and health providers, and extensive web links.
Note: Resources available in Spanish.

Lesbian

☐ Kathy's Group
kathysgroupinc@juno.com
(888) 5KATHYS

Kathy's Group provides supportive resources for lesbians and their families who have been affected by cancer.

☐ **The Lesbian Community Cancer Project**
www.lccp.org
4753 N. Broadway, Suite 602
Chicago, IL 60640-4907
(773) 561-4662

Gives support, information, education, advocacy, and direct services to lesbians and women living with cancer and their families. The pamphlet *Lesbians and Cancer* provides early detection information.

Note: Resources available in Spanish.

Lesbians with Breast Cancer Keep in Touch
To subscribe: LBCKIT@yahoogroups.com

Online email support group for lesbians with breast cancer and their partners. Its aim is to get women talking to each other across geographical boundaries and for women to chip in their opinions on treatment, fears, and relationships.

☐ **Mautner Project for Lesbians with Cancer**
www.mautnerproject.org
1707 L Street NW, Suite 500
Washington, DC 20036
(202) 332-5536

A volunteer organization dedicated to helping lesbians with cancer, as well as their partners and caregivers. The pamphlet *Lesbians and Cancer* provides early detection information and addresses issues for lesbians.

Note: Resources available in Spanish.

Rose Penski, **by Ros Perry** (Naiad Press, 1989).

A novel about a lesbian, Adelle, and her lover, Rose, going through diagnosis and initial treatment of breast cancer. The reader will find hints on managing breast cancer, enlightenment on female-to-female sex, and fine suggestions for good eating.

Seattle Lesbian Cancer Project
www.slcp.org
1122 E. Pike Street, No. 1333
Seattle, WA 98122
(206) 286-0166

Seattle-based grassroots organization providing advocacy, education, and referrals, with an emphasis on the medically underserved.

*Wendy's Hope: Reaching Out to Lesbians with Cancer
and Other Life-Threatening Diseases*
City of Hope
1055 Wilshire Boulevard, 12th Floor
Los Angeles, CA 90017
(310) 798-9085
Wendy's Hope marks the first partnership of its kind between a national cancer center and members of the gay and lesbian community. Offers education, assistance, and support groups.

Native American

American Indian Women's Health Demonstration Project
San Francisco, Calif.
(415) 865-0964
Health and wellness education program for Native American women.

Native American Women's Health Education Resource Center
www.nativeshop.org/nawherc.html
PO Box 572
Lake Andes, SD 57356-0572
(605) 487-7072
Reservation-based resource center; provides comprehensive women's health services and education and technical assistance to other groups.

Susan G. Komen Breast Cancer Foundation:
Native American Women and Breast Cancer
www.breastcancerinfo.com/bhealth/html/native_american.html
Information for Native American women on the risk of developing breast cancer is provided on this webpage. The fact sheet discusses the relatively high mortality rates for Native Americans diagnosed with breast cancer and stresses the importance of screening.

HORMONAL THERAPY

☐ **NABCO Information Packet.**
Available at nabcoinfo@aol.com or call (888) 80-NABCO.
Packet of relevant journal articles and fact sheets on hormonal therapy.

☐ *Questions and Answers About Tamoxifen* (1994).
Call (800) 4-CANCER.
A fact sheet on tamoxifen (Nolvadex) and its side effects.

Tamoxifen and Breast Cancer, **by Michael W. DeGregorio and
Valeria J. Wiebe** (University Press, 1999).
Book presents a balanced discussion of the diagnosis of breast cancer
and the risks, benefits, and limitations of treatment alternatives, particularly
tamoxifen. There is helpful information regarding the latest developments
in the use of tamoxifen, especially the results of the Breast Cancer Prevention Trial.

HOSPICE AND FAMILY CARE

Home Care Guide for Advanced Cancer. Available at www.acponline.
org/public/homecare or through the American College of Physicians, 190
N. Independence Mall West, Philadelphia, PA 19106-1572, (800) 523-
1546, ext. 2600.
The American College of Physicians' online guide for family, friends,
and hospice workers caring for patients with advanced cancer at home.

Hospice Foundation of America
www.hospicefoundation.org
20001 S Street NW, Suite 300
Washington, DC 20009
(202) 638-5419
Services include: guide to locate hospice services, low-cost brochures
and videos, searchable end-of-life database, links to related websites, an extensive reading list, and teleconferences.

National Family Caregivers Association
www.nfcacares.org
c/o National Family Counseling Association
10400 Connecticut Avenue, No. 500
Kensington, MD 20895
(800) 896-3650
Offers information, education, support, public education, and advocacy
to address the common needs of family caregivers.

National Hospice and Palliative Care Organization
www.nhpco.org
1700 Diagonal Road, Suite 300
Alexandria, VA 22314
(703) 837-1500
Offers excellent resources for finding hospice resources, if your local
hospital is unable to help. Many professional resources are listed as well.
Note: Resources available in Spanish.

R. A. Bloch Cancer Foundation
www.blochcancer.org
4400 Main Street
Kansas City, MO 64111
(800) 433-0464
Matches newly diagnosed cancer patients with trained, home-based
volunteers who have been treated for the same type of cancer. Also distributes informational materials, including a multidisciplinary list of institutions that offer second opinions.
Note: Resources available in Spanish.

INSPIRATIONAL READING

*Examining Myself: One Woman's Story of Breast Cancer Treatment and
Recovery,* **by Musa Mayer** (Faber and Faber, 1994).
Brilliant first-person account of a woman dealing with breast cancer.
The narrative flows smoothly from personal experience and intense emo-
tion to important, accurate technical information. Mayer describes diagnosis,
surgery, chemotherapy, and recovery as well as feelings of fear, uncertainty,

self-blame, depression, and shifts in relationships that most women with breast cancer experience.

Kitchen Table Wisdom, **by Rachel Naomi Remen, M.D.** (Riverhead Books, 1997).

It is impossible to walk away from this book unchanged. Dr. Remen addresses healing by sharing heartfelt short stories.

Straight from the Heart: Letters of Hope and Inspiration from Survivors of Breast Cancer, **by Ina Yalof** (Kensington Books, 1997).

A carefully compiled collection of nearly 100 letters from women who have been diagnosed with breast cancer. Some are newly diagnosed; others have survived for decades. They're women from all walks of life, all ages, and all backgrounds with a common will to live.

ADVOCACY AND POLITICS

The Activist Cancer Patient: How to Take Charge of Your Treatment, **by Beverly Zakarian** (Wiley, 1996).

Zakarian, a cancer survivor, has written a moving, inspirational, and practical aid for cancer patients. While empowerment is the main theme, the book is also a step-by-step guide on how to improve your odds of surviving cancer. It teaches people in the midst of crisis how to become activists for their own most effective cancer treatment and how to gain access to the newest therapies, and suggests how they can apply what they've learned to the public arena.

☐ **Breast Cancer Action**
www.bcaction.org
55 New Montgomery, Suite 624
San Francisco, CA 94105
(415) 243-9301

A grassroots group committed to serving as a catalyst for the prevention and cure of breast cancer through education and advocacy, through helping to refocus research on detecting the causes of breast cancer, and through empowering women and men to have a voice in decisions about their diagnosis and treatment.

Note: Resources available in Spanish.

Linda Creed Breast Cancer Foundation
http://www.lindacreed.org
Medical Tower Building
255 S. 17th Street, Suite 905
Philadelphia, PA 19103
(215) 545-0800
Committed to empowering women and their families to practice breast health, foster the healing process, and establish a public agenda for prevention and cure.

☐ **Los Angeles Breast Cancer Alliance (LABCA)**
www.labca.com
2125 Arizona Avenue, Suite 102
Santa Monica, CA 90404
(310) 453-1046
A grassroots, nonprofit organization dedicated to helping in the eradication of breast cancer through advocacy, education, and community involvement. Concerned survivors and supporters formed LABCA in 1992.

☐ **Men Against Breast Cancer**
www.menagainstbreastcancer.org
2379 Lewis Avenue
Rockville, MD 20851
(866) 547-MABC
A national organization that encourages men to actively participate in the fight for a cure.

☐ **National Breast Cancer Coalition (NBCC)**
www.natlbcc.org
1707 L Street NW, Suite 1060
Washington, DC 20036
(202) 296-7477
Coalition of over 500 groups involves women with the disease and those who care about them in changing public policy as it relates to progress against breast cancer. The NBCC welcomes individuals and organizations as members.

□ **One in Nine/Long Island Breast Cancer Action Coalition**
www.1in9.org
PO Box 729
Baldwin, NY 11510
(516) 357-9622

One in Nine/Long Island Breast Cancer Action Coalition actively keeps the breast cancer epidemic in the forefront of public awareness, promotes legislative and environmental issues beneficial to finding a cause and a cure for breast cancer, educates constituents about the latest advances in resources, research, and treatment, and obtains funding for research.

Patient No More: The Politics of Breast Cancer, by Sharon Batt (Gynergy Books, 1994).

Sharon Batt goes behind all the feel-good, superficial cheerleading hype so common in books written by survivors to get at the "real" story behind the "breast cancer industry." You will never look at breast cancer the same way after you read this book.

FINANCIAL ASSISTANCE

□ **AirLifeLine Midwest**
www.airlifelinemidwest.org/index2.htm
Suite 302, Byerly Terminal
Greater Peoria Regional Airport
6100 W. Dirksen Parkway
Peoria, IL 61607
(800) 822-7972

A private, nonprofit organization that flies qualified patients to treatment centers nationwide.

□ **American Cancer Society**
www.cancer.org
(800) ACS-2345

The office in your area can provide information on local sources of financial assistance. Check your telephone directory for the number.

Note: Resources available in Spanish.

☐ **Cancer Care, Inc.**
www.cancercare.org
(800) 813-HOPE
Toll-free counseling line staffed with trained social workers that can suggest referrals for financial assistance. The AVONCares program at Cancer Care, Inc., provides financial assistance for diagnostic and support services.

☐ **Cancer Fund of America**
http://cfoa.org
(800) 578-5284
Provides direct aid to financially challenged patients in the form of canned goods, medical supplies, and other necessary staples.

☐ **Corporate Angel Network, Inc.**
www.corpangelnetwork.org
Westchester County Airport
1 Loop Road
White Plains, NY 10604
(914) 328-1313
Free service that flies qualified patients with confirmed appointments to treatment centers.

☐ **Hill-Burton Free Care Program**
www.hrsa.dhhs.gov/osp/dfcr
(800) 638-0742 or (800) 492-0359 in Maryland
This national government agency provides referrals for free medical care at participating medical facilities, mostly hospitals, and helps low-income individuals pay their medical bills.

☐ **The Medicine Program**
http://themedicineprogram.com
(573) 996-7300, Mon.–Fri., 8 A.M.–5 P.M., EST
This national nonprofit organization provides free prescriptions for those who qualify.

☐ *The National Financial Resource Guidebook for Patients* (Patient Advocate Foundation, 1999). Available at www.patientadvocate.org or Patient Advocate Foundation, 753 Thimble Shoals Boulevard, Suite B, Newport

News, VA 23606, (800) 532-5274. One state directory is free; complete book is $19.95.

This valuable resource provides listings of federal and state resources for obtaining financial assistance for housing, transportation, utilities, medical payments, and insurance deductibles.

Pharmaceutical Breast Cancer Patient Assistant Program

www.phrma.org

1100 Fifteenth Street NW

Washington, DC 20005

(202) 835-3400

Check the website of the Pharmaceutical Research and Manufacturers of America (PhRMA) for information about selected company reimbursement assistance programs for oncology-related products. Eligibility requirements and application procedures vary with each program, and a physician or nurse on the breast cancer patient's behalf best accesses these programs. Some companies offer free products for women who are uninsured and can demonstrate financial need.

INSURANCE COVERAGE

□ Agency for Healthcare Research and Quality

www.ahcpr.gov/consumer

(301) 594-1364

Publishes guidelines on choosing health plans and health insurance choices. Publications are available free for viewing on their website.

Note: Information available in Spanish.

The Alliance of Claims Assistance Professionals

www.claims.org

873 Brentwood Drive

West Chicago, IL 60185-3743

(877) 275-8765

Offers assistance in getting insurers to pay for experimental treatments, as well as other reimbursement and billing problems.

□ **American Association of Retired Persons (AARP)**
www.aarp.org
(800) 424-3410

A resource for problems with health insurance companies and for help navigating the health care system. Provides free publications for caregivers and for those over age 50.

□ *A Cancer Survivor's Almanac.* Call (888) 937-6227.

Contains useful information about insurance coverage. From the National Coalition for Cancer Survivorship.

□ *Cancer Treatments Your Insurance Should Cover* (April 1995). Available at www.assoc-cancer-ctrs.org/ or order from the Association of Community Cancer Centers, 11600 Nebel Street, Suite 201, Rockville, MD 20852, (301) 984-9496.

This 8-page brochure describes standard and investigational treatments that should be covered, and what to do if reimbursement is denied.

Center for Patient Advocacy's Insurance-Help Hotline
(800) 846-7444

Can serve as an alternative to litigation for patients who are denied coverage.

□ *The Consumer's Guide to Disability Insurance* (1995).
(202) 824-1600.

A comprehensive 12-page guide to understanding disability insurance from the Health Insurance Association of America.

□ *The Consumer's Guide to Medicare Supplement Insurance* (1995).
(202) 824-1600.

Instructions on using private insurance to supplement Medicare for maximum coverage from the Health Insurance Association of America.

Medicaid
www.hcfa.gov/medicaid

A federal-state partnership medical insurance program based on financial need. To receive Medicaid, your income and assets must be below a certain level. It covers hospital care, physician's fees, prescription drugs,

home care, and many other services. In addition, the Community Alternatives Program for Disabled Adults (CAP/DA) provides a package of services to allow adults who qualify for nursing facility care to remain in their
private residences. In order to qualify, you must be a U.S. resident. See your
local social services office to apply.

Medicare
www.medicare.gov
(800) MEDICARE ([800] 633-4227)

A government-sponsored medical insurance program, usually for people
who are aged 65 or older. People who have been disabled and receiving Social Security Disability payments for 24 months are also eligible. Benefits
vary from person to person. Medicare provides basic health coverage but it
doesn't pay for all of your health expenses.

Medicare is divided into two parts:

Part A: pays for hospital care, home health care, hospice care, and care
in certified nursing facilities. It is free.

Part B: covers diagnostic studies, physician's service, medical equipment
used at home, and ambulance transportation.

Medigap: If you are on Medicare, you may be able to add more coverage with a Medigap policy or a Medicare HMO. Insurance carriers
offer different plans. Check with them to get more information.

□ The National Insurance Consumer Helpline
(800) 942-4242

A hotline that answers consumer questions and offers problem-solving
support and printed materials, including information on life and property
casualty insurance. Open Mon.–Fri., 8:00 A.M.–8:00 P.M., EST.

□ *Questions Women with Breast Cancer Frequently Ask about Health Insurance Benefits.* Available at www.med.jhu.edu/breastcenter/treatment/
choice/questions.htm. Informative webpage from the Breast Center at
Johns Hopkins. Call (800) 998-7542.

This pamphlet from the U.S. Department of Labor, Pension, and Welfare Benefits Administration, describes the Health Insurance Portability and
Accountability Act (HIPAA) of 1996. This service also publishes *Questions
and Answers: Recent Changes in Healthcare Law,* a summary guide to the HIPAA.

□ *Your Medicare Handbook.* Available from Health Care Finance Administration (HLFA), 6325 Security Boulevard, Baltimore, MD 21207, (800) 638-6833.

Medicare beneficiaries should obtain this pamphlet from the federal agency that administers Medicare.

LEGAL ISSUES

□ *The Americans with Disabilities Act: Protection for Cancer Patients against Employment Discrimination* (4585, 1993). Call (800) ACS-2345.

Brochure defines the ADA law by describing employment rights of the cancer patient.

Be Prepared—The Complete Financial, Legal, and Practical Guide for Living with a Life-Challenging Condition, by **David S. Landay** (St. Martin's Press, 2000).

Be Prepared is an incredible compilation of useful and practical information for anyone dealing with serious illness. Not only provides the tools to evaluate a situation realistically but also points out many issues that you may not even think of.

□ *Cancer: Your Job, Insurance and the Law* (4585-PS, 1987). Available at www.cancer.org or call (800) ACS-2345.

This 6-page pamphlet from the ACS summarizes cancer patients' legal rights and gives complaint procedure instructions.

□ **Judges and Lawyers Breast Cancer Alert**
50 King Street, Suite 6D
New York, NY 10014
Confidential hotline for judges, lawyers, and law students who have been diagnosed with breast cancer.

Patient Advocate Foundation (PAF)
www.patientadvocate.org
(800) 532-5274
Provides education, legal counseling, and referrals to cancer patients and survivors concerning managed care, insurance, financial issues, job discrim-

ination, and debt crisis matters. Also publishes the consumer publication *The Managed Care Answer Guide* (1997), a reference handbook for cancer patients insured by managed care plans.

□ **Social Security Administration**
(800) 772-1213
You may be eligible for Supplemental Security Income (SSI) and/or Social Security benefits. While receiving SSI, you could also be eligible for food stamps and Medicaid. For information, ask your hospital social worker or call the Social Security Administration.

□ *State Laws Relating to Breast Cancer* (CDC, March 1998). Available at www.cdc.gov or call (770) 488-4751 or (800) 813-HOPE.
The Centers for Disease Control and Prevention has published a summary of statutes across the country related to breast cancer. Available from the CDC or Cancer Care, Inc., based in New York City.

□ **Volunteer Legal Service Program–Cancer Legal Services Project**
jseldon@sfbar.org
Bar Association of San Francisco
465 California Street, No. 1100
San Francisco, CA 94104
(415) 989-1616
Provides free and low-cost legal services for low-income people with breast cancer. Services include wills, powers of attorney for health care and property management, insurance issues, and guardianships. Clients are screened and then referred to a private attorney who will volunteer services for free consultation and representation.
Note: Interpreter services available by prior arrangement.

LYMPH NODES

□ **Sentinel Node Biopsy**
www.nsabp.pitt.edu
(412) 330-4600
The National Surgical Adjuvant Breast and Bowel Project, a cooperative group, conducts clinical trials, including studies on this innovative technique.

MAGAZINES, NEWSLETTERS, AND NEWS SOURCES

☐ *Artemis.* Available at www.med.jhu.edu/breastcenter/artemis.

Monthly e-zine from Johns Hopkins Hospital. Recent breast cancer–related topics included: "How Informed Is Informed Consent?" "Patients Don't Follow Cancer Pain Prescriptions," "Assessing the Benefits of Support Groups," and "Getting Rid of Radiation Tattoos."

☐ **Breastcancer.net**

www.breastcancer.net

This news site supplies up-to-the-minute information on breast cancer topics in recent and archived news articles. Late-breaking stories on breast cancer are posted on the home page. Activate the link "Newsroom" and you can reach 1,500 additional articles. Support and treatment are other useful links on the site, and there is a link to other important Internet sites relating to breast cancer.

☐ **Breast Link**

www.breastlink.com/blink/plsql/homepage

Provided by the Breast Cancer Care and Research Fund, this resource includes recent medical news, an online bookstore, a description of the Breast Cancer Care and Research Fund, and a search tool allowing searches for articles by category or therapy. Consumer resources on digesting science news are provided, along with explanations of important parts of a scientific study and suggestions for reviewing technical journal articles.

Note: Resources available in Spanish.

☐ **Cancer News on the Net**

www.cancernews.com

Cancer News on the Net features original articles about many types of cancer. It also links to other cancer information sites.

☐ **CancerWeb**

http://infoventures.com/CANCER

CancerWeb contains the *CancerWeb Report,* a monthly publication alerting you to the latest information appearing in recent issues of cancer-related research and medical journals, original summaries of the non–NLM-derived portion of *CANCERLIT,* links to other cancer-related resources, mail from readers, and a calendar of meetings and conferences.

Coping Magazine. Available at Copingmag@aol.com or Media America, Inc., 2019 N. Carothers, Franklin, TN 37064, (617) 790-2400.
A bimonthly magazine for cancer patients and survivors.

In Touch. Available at www.intouchlive.com/journals/intouch/home.htm.
A magazine dedicated to cancer prevention and treatment. The website offers a link to receive two free introductory issues.

MAMM Magazine: Women, Cancer and Community. Available at www.mamm.com or POZ Publishing, 349 W. 12th Street, New York, NY 10014-1721, (888) 901-MAMM.
MAMM Covers issues helpful to women who have been diagnosed with breast and reproductive cancer and their partners and families.

NABCO News. Available at www.nabco.org or 9 E. 37th Street, 10th Floor, New York, NY 10016, (888) 80-NABCO.
National Alliance of Breast Cancer Organizations (NABCO) publishes a quarterly newsletter, *NABCO News,* and the annual *Breast Cancer Resource List.*

Surviving! Available at www-radonc.stanford.edu/surviving.html or Department of Radiation Oncology, Stanford University Medical Center, Division of Radiation Therapy, Room A035, Stanford, CA 94305-5304, (650) 723-7881.
Surviving! is a newsletter written and created by cancer patients, for the benefit of cancer patients and their friends and families.

MASTECTOMY, LUMPECTOMY, BREAST RECONSTRUCTION, AND IMPLANTS

☐ **American Society of Plastic and Reconstructive Surgeons**
www.plasticsurgery.org for additional information.
(800) 635-0635

Call for referrals to a plastic surgeon for corrective or reconstructive procedures, and a list of several local board-certified plastic surgeons will be mailed to you.

Breast Implants: Everything You Need to Know, by Nancy Bruning (Hunter House, 1995).

According to Amazon.com, "This edition discusses current research on the relationship between breast implants and disease; hardening, leaking, and rupture of implants; and relevant court decisions. The author also discusses the newest implant techniques and guidelines for having implants removed or replaced."

□ *Breast Reconstruction after Mastectomy* (4630, American Cancer Society, 2000). Call (800) ACS-2345.

This 20-page pamphlet from the ACS describes types of surgery, with photographs and drawings, and gives answers to commonly asked questions as well as a glossary of terms.

□ **The Council for Breast Reconstruction Awareness and Education**
(800) 327-1168

A consumer hotline, offering educational resources about breast reconstruction.

□ **FDA (Food and Drug Administration) Breast Implant Information Line**
(800) 532-4440

Answers consumer and professional inquiries about breast implants; assists in registering complaints and accessing implant registries. Established in 1992.

□ **Imaginis.net: Lumpectomy**
www.imaginis.com/breasthealth/lumpectomy.asp

Provided by Imaginis.net, this site provides an overview of the lumpectomy procedure, with information offered on determining candidacy for lumpectomy, the lumpectomy procedure, radiation therapy after lumpectomy, and auxiliary node dissection.

☐ *Implants: An Information Update* (U.S. Food and Drug Administration). Call (800) 532-4440.

Contains information about silicone gel–filled and saline-filled breast implants for reconstruction and augmentation. Covers issues such as FDA regulation, scientific studies, alternatives to breast implants, and answers to frequently asked questions.

☐ *Mastectomy: A Treatment for Breast Cancer* (87-658, National Cancer Institute, 1997). Call (800) 4-CANCER.

Information about different types of breast surgery.

☐ **RENU Breast Reconstruction Counseling**
Einstein Medical Center
5501 Old York Road
Philadelphia, PA 19141
(215) 456-7387

A support program staffed by trained volunteers who have had post-mastectomy reconstruction. Hotline counseling and written materials are available.

Show Me: A Photo Collection of Breast Cancer Survivors' Lumpectomies, Mastectomies, Reconstructions and Thoughts on Body Image. Available at SusanLoveMD.com or Penn State Geisinger Health System Women's Center, Box 850, Code H306, Hershey, PA 17033, (717) 531-5867.

This amazing resource, created by a breast cancer support group, shows what your body will look like after different breast surgeries.

☐ **Womens Health and Cancer Rights Act of 1998.** For questions and answers about the Act visit www.dol.gov/pwba/pubs/womhlth.htm. For a copy of the law, contact the U.S. Department of Labor, Pension and Welfare Benefits Administration, (415) 975-4600.

States that women who are eligible for mastectomy benefits under group coverage and who elect breast reconstruction in conjunction with surgery are eligible to receive coverage for reconstruction on the breast on which the mastectomy has been performed; surgery and reconstruction on the other breast to produce a symmetrical appearance; and prosthesis and treatment for any physical complication, including lymphedema.

METASTASIS

Advanced Breast Cancer: A Guide to Living with Metastatic Disease, **by Musa Mayer** (Patient Centered Guides, 1998).

This updated, retitled edition of the author's 1997 *Holding Tight, Letting Go* helps women lead everyday lives while coping with advanced disease. Includes information on treatment options, managing side effects and pain, finding support, and handling emotional issues along with personal stories of men and women living with metastatic breast cancer.

Cancer in Two Voices, **by Sandra Butler and Barbara Rosenblum** (contributor) (Bookpeople, 1996).

When Barbara Rosenblum was diagnosed with advanced breast cancer in 1985, she was the first among her friends to get sick. Rosenblum and her lesbian partner, Sandra Butler, committed themselves to making the most of their remaining years and wrote this heartwarming book.

☐ **Metastatic Breast Cancer Website**
www.bcmets.org
An online source for information about metastatic cancer created by members of bcmets, an online support community.

☐ *NABCO Information Packet*
(888) 80-NABCO
Relevant journal articles and fact sheets on recurrence and advanced breast cancer.

POSTSURGERY PRODUCTS AND RESOURCES

American Hair Loss Council
www.ahlc.org
165 N. Village Avenue, Suite 128
Rockville Center, NY 11570
(877) HAIR-USA
Provides a hotline for information on hair loss.

Becoming, Inc.
(800) 980-9085
Sells lingerie, workout wear, swimsuits, wigs, breast forms, and accessories.

Best Look Forward (Graduate Hospital, 1991). Available at The Graduate Hospital Cancer Program, 1840 South Street, Philadelphia, PA 19146, (215) 893-7298.
In this 30-minute videotape, make-up artists and hairdressers give advice and demonstrations, including on eyebrows and lashes. $45.

Edith Imre Foundation for Loss of Hair
30 W. 57th Street, 2nd Floor
New York, NY 10019
Wig hotline (212) 765-8397
Provides counseling and support as well as a selection of appropriate wigs. Accepts Medicaid.

Ladies' First Choice
www.wvi.com/~ladies1
(800) 300-3940 or (800) 497-8285
Ladies First offers after-breast-surgery and immediate-postmastectomy products designed by a breast cancer survivor.

☐ *Look Good . . . Feel Better: Caring for Yourself Inside and Out* (CTFA Foundation, 1988). Call (800) 395-LOOK.
In LGFB Programs 16-minute video for cancer patients undergoing chemotherapy and radiation therapy, women candidly discuss their experiences, and beauty professionals review ways to look and feel better during treatment, including makeup, nail care, and wigs.
Note: Instructional sessions in Spanish available in some locations run by the ACS.

Maintaining a Positive Image with Breast Cancer Surgery. Available at Johanna's on Call to Mend Esteem, 199 New Scotland Avenue, Albany, NY 12208, (518) 482-4178.
Videotape covering prosthetic, lingerie, and swimsuit choices following breast cancer surgery.

Ramy Beauty Therapy

www.ramybeautytherapy.com

(888) 550-RAMY

Also sold at: Bergdorf Goodman, New York, (212) 753-7300, and Skin Solutions, Atlanta, Ga., (404) 495-9099. Makeup developed by a cancer survivor; includes *Miracle Brow,* a natural-looking eyebrow maker and *Alive* blush.

□ **Tender Loving Care (TLC) Catalog.** Call (800) 850-9455.

Catalog from the American Cancer Society features helpful items like bras and hats for female cancer survivors. Medicare reimbursement for products is available.

□ **Women's Healthcare Educational Network, Inc.**

(800) 991-8877

Call for a list of 78 member shops specializing in postsurgery products.

□ **Y-ME Prosthesis and Wig Bank**

www.y-me.org

212 W. Van Buren Street, 4th Floor

Chicago, IL 60607

(800) 221-2141

This coalition of over 500 groups involves women with the disease and those who care about them in changing public policy as it relates to progress against breast cancer. The NBCC welcomes individuals and organizations as members. Y-ME National Breast Cancer Organization maintains a prosthesis and wig bank for women in financial need. If the appropriate size is available, Y-ME will mail a wig and/or breast prosthesis anywhere in the country. The organization's hotline is staffed with breast cancer survivors and is a 24-hour service. A nominal handling fee is requested.

PREGNANCY AND BREAST CANCER

□ **Pregnancy after Breast Cancer**

www.moffitt.usf.edu/pubs/ccj/v6n3/article6.htm

Hosted by the H. Lee Moffitt Cancer Center and Research Institute, this site features a full-text article on pregnancy after breast cancer. Historical studies and population-based reports of women bearing children after treatment for breast cancer are discussed. The needs for future studies, along with advice to current patients, are also provided.

☐ *CancerNet PDQ: Breast Cancer and Pregnancy.* Available at www. cancer.gov/cancer_information/doc_pdq.aspx?viewid=51DC247F-9F08-4A0C-A0A2-42B94848FC74.

A PDQ on breast cancer treatment during pregnancy is featured on this web page. Information on diagnosis in pregnant women, as well as staging modified to avoid radiation exposure, is provided. Treatment options by stage are outlined briefly. Lactation, as well as the effect of cancer on the fetus, are discussed.

☐ **Pregnant with Cancer Support Group**
www.pregnantwithcancer.org
PO Box 1243
Buffalo, NY 14220
(800) 743–6724, ext. 308

This national organization was created to provide support for women who are facing a diagnosis of cancer while pregnant. This group will match a new patient with someone who once faced cancer while pregnant.

PREVENTION AND RISK REDUCTION

The Breast Cancer Prevention Program, by Samuel S. Epstein, David Steinman, and Suzanne Levert (Hungry Minds, 1998).

This book contains valuable information that the cancer establishment will not tell you about. Dr. Epstein's message: Cut your exposure to toxins and strengthen your own immune system so that you reduce your risk of ever getting cancer; this book will drastically change the way we see breast cancer prevention.

Cancer Therapy: The Independent Consumer's Guide to Non-Toxic Treatments and Prevention, by Ralph Moss (Equinox Press, 1993).

This thorough guide is a must-read for cancer patients and their families seeking treatment options. Moss gives an excellent overview of many alternative treatments, although some of the material is no longer current.

☐ **Centers for Disease Control and Prevention (CDC)**

www.cdc.gov

The CDC website provides publications, travelers' health information, statistics, and training, employment, and other information.

Note: Resources available in Spanish.

Stopping Cancer Before It Starts: The American Institute for Cancer Research's Program for Cancer Prevention (Golden Book, 1999).

This book provides a good insight into the role that various factors, such as diet, exercise, and obesity, play in cancer prevention. It combines solid information with practical ideas for making lifestyle changes for lower cancer risk.

RECOVERING/SURVIVING

☐ **Living Beyond Breast Cancer (LBBC)**

www.lbbc.org

10 E. Athens Avenue, Suite 204

Ardmore, PA 19003

(610) 645-4567

A nonprofit educational organization founded in 1992 by Marisa C. Weiss, M.D., a radiation oncologist; created to address the physical, social, emotional, legal, and financial issues women face after they have completed their primary treatment for breast cancer. Programs include semiannual large-scale educational conferences, a quarterly educational newsletter, outreach to medically underserved women, a consumer-focused educational pamphlet, the Paula A. Seidman Library and Resource Center, Young Survivors group, the Survivors' Helpline, and a website.

☐ **National Coalition for Cancer Survivorship**

www.cansearch.org

1010 Wayne Avenue, 5th Floor

Silver Spring, MD 20910

(877) NCCS-YES (622-7937) or (877) TOOLS-4-U (866-5748)

A national network of independent groups and individuals concerned about survivorship and sources of support for cancer patients and their families. It is a clearinghouse for information and advocates for cancer survivors.

☐ **Project Survive**

Health.psy.uab.edu/survive

Researchers at the University of Alabama created this website with free group therapy and bulletin boards for survivors.

☐ **Reach To Recovery**

www.cancer.org

(800) ACS-2345

An 8-week exercise and early and later support program for women who have had surgery for breast cancer, sponsored by the American Cancer Society. The exercises are specifically designed for the special requirements of recuperating patients. Bras and prosthesis are also offered.

Uplift: Secrets from the Sisterhood of Breast Cancer Survivors, **by Barbara Delinsky** (Pocket Books, 2001).

Delinsky, a survivor of breast cancer, presents inspirational snippets from more than 300 women sharing breast cancer tips and experiences. Every woman should read this book, whether she is a survivor, just diagnosed, or a woman with empathy for what others think, feel, and experience during their healing.

The Victoria's Secret Catalog Never Stops Coming: And Other Lessons I Learned from Breast Cancer, **by Jennie Nash** (Scribner's, 2001).

Beautiful story of one woman who had the courage to take notes while she was sick with breast cancer and who shares her experience and lessons learned.

SELECTING A DOCTOR/ BREAST CANCER SPECIALIST

☐ **National Alliance of Breast Cancer Organizations (NABCO)**

www.nabco.org

9 E. 37th Street, 10th Floor

New York, NY 10016

(888) 80-NABCO

An excellent resource for finding board-certified surgical breast specialist or surgical oncologist referrals.

☐ **The American Board of Medical Specialists**
(800) 776-2378
Can verify a physician's board certification by specialty and year, and will refer callers to local board-certified doctors.

☐ **American Society of Clinical Oncology**
www.asco.org
(703) 299-0150
Your doctor can also contact the ASCO or to be referred to local surgical oncologists who are ASCO members.

☐ **National Cancer Institute (NCI)**
www.nci.nih.gov
(800) 4-CANCER
Call NCIs Cancer Information Service for the names of NCI-affiliated treatment centers in your state. If none of these centers is conveniently located, call the department of surgery at the nearest one and ask for a local referral.

☐ **State Health Departments**
Many state health departments now maintain a "Consumer Information" section of their websites that includes an updated, alphabetical listing of state physicians who have been cited for professional misconduct.

☐ *Talking with Your Doctor* (4638-CC, American Cancer Society, 1997). Call (800) ACS-2345.
Six-page pamphlet with suggestions for effective doctor/patient communication.

SEXUALITY

☐ *Breast Cancer and Sexuality* (Cancer Care, 1998). Call (800) 813-HOPE
Pamphlet from Cancer Care discusses sexuality, intimacy, and menopausal symptoms in an honest and supportive manner.

Good Vibrations

www.goodvibes.com

(800) 289-8423 for free catalog

Whether you're looking for sexual information or inspiration, Good Vibrations is a great authority on toys and educational resources.

No Less a Woman: Femininity, Sexuality and Breast Cancer, **by Deborah Hobler Kahane** (Hunter House, 1995).

This insightful book is much more than just a collection of different women's individual stories of breast cancer and the decisions they made—it talks about confronting cancer, making choices, finding support, and moving forward.

☐ *Sexuality and Cancer: For the Woman Who Has Cancer and Her Partner* (American Cancer Society, 1999). Call (800) ACS-2345.

A 64-page pamphlet that gives information about cancer and sexuality in areas that might concern the patient and her partner.

Sexuality and Fertility After Cancer, by Leslie R. Schover, Ph.D. (Wiley, 1997).

If the shock of a cancer diagnosis doesn't wreak havoc on your sex life, the treatments probably will. This book offers lots of suggestions for maintaining and/or improving intimacy and sex during and after cancer.

SUPPORT AND RESOURCES FOR PATIENTS, FAMILY MEMBERS, AND CAREGIVERS

☐ **Arm-in-Arm**

(410) 494-0083

A breast cancer support group created to promote the physical and emotional well-being of women with breast cancer by providing friendship, support, and understanding. A member of NBCC and NABCO.

☐ **Breast Cancer Advocate**

421 Woodbine Lane

Danville, CA 94526

(925) 820-1569 (24-hour answering machine)

A consultant who offers counseling to breast cancer patients over the phone and will visit the doctor with patients for the first appointment (if local). Brochure available. Services are free.

Breast Cancer Listserv

www.bclist.org

Since the spring of 1994, the Breast Cancer List has been available on the Internet for women and men who have breast cancer, their families and friends, medical and other caregivers, researchers, students, and other concerned people. This important resource takes the form of email postings routed through a central distributing address to the in box at each subscriber's email program. Subscription to this discussion list is free.

□ **Breast Friends**

(888) 718-3523

Take it from women who've been there—this round-the-clock support line run by breast cancer survivors offers invaluable comfort, support, and information.

□ **Cancer Hope Network**

www.cancerhopenetwork.org

Two North Road

Chester, NJ 07930

(877) HOPENET

Cancer Hope Network matches patients with cancer with trained volunteers who have themselves undergone a similar experience.

□ **Cancer Information and Counseling Line (CICL)**
(a service of the AMC Cancer Research Center)

www.amc.org

(800) 525-3777, Cancer Information and Counseling Line (CICL), 8:30 A.M.–5:00 P.M., EST

The CICL, part of the Psychosocial Program of the AMC Cancer Research Center, is a toll-free telephone service for cancer patients, their family members and friends, cancer survivors, and the general public. Professional counselors provide up-to-date medical information, emotional support through short-term counseling, and resource referrals to callers nationwide.

Individuals may also submit questions about cancer and request resources via email.

☐ **The Cancer Wellness Center/The Barbara Kassel Brotman House**
215 Revere Drive
Northbrook, IL 50062
(708) 509-9595
Offers free emotional support on its 24-hour hotline and through support groups, relaxation groups, educational workshops, and library.

☐ *How to Find Resources in Your Own Community If You Have Cancer.*
Go to http://cis.nci.nih.gov/fact/8_9.htm.
This helpful website from the National Cancer Institute is a good starting point for finding local resources. Includes the categories Information on Cancer, Counseling, Medical Treatment Decisions, Prevention and Early Detection, Home Health Care, Hospice Care, Rehabilitation, Advocacy, Financial, Housing/Lodging, and Childrens Services.

☐ **Johns Hopkins Breast Center**
www.med.jhu.edu/breastcenter
601 N. Caroline Street
Baltimore, MD 21287
(410) 614-2853
A comprehensive, multidisciplinary breast care program, offering a full spectrum of clinical and support services, from screening and diagnosis to treatment and counseling. The Center provides innovative, integrated, high-quality, and cost-effective care.

- *Easing the Hurt:* An Online Support Group for Johns Hopkins Oncology Center Patients Experiencing Cancer Pain; facilitator: Kathy Smolinski, LCSW-C, (410) 955-5637.
- *Reaching Out to Families at Home:* An Online Support Group for Caregivers of Patients at the Johns Hopkins Oncology Center; facilitator: Alice Rainess, LCSW-C, (410) 955-8973.

For registration and information about these online groups, please do not hesitate to contact the group facilitators. All participants need to be pre-registered. For more information or flyers, contact Kim at bellki@jhmi.edu.

☐ **medGrasp—For the Patient, By the Patient**

www.breast-cancer-support.com

A breast cancer "community site" where users can share experiences, read medical postings, consult a medical dictionary, chat online, and browse relevant health news.

☐ **SHARE Self-Help for Women With Breast Cancer and Ovarian Cancer**

www.noah.cuny.edu/share.html

(212) 382-2111 (English) or (212) 719-4454 (Spanish)

A self-help organization for women with breast or ovarian cancer. Breast cancer survivors provide emotional support, resources, and information about breast cancer, including services for men with breast cancer. Hotline available Mon.–Fri., 9:30 A.M.–5:00 P.M., EST.

Note: Hotline services available in Spanish and Russian.

☐ **SusanLoveMD.com**

www.susanlovemd.com

Provides breast cancer content, chat, and community for baby boomer women.

☐ **The Wellness Community**

www.wellness-community.org

35 E. Seventh Street

Suite 412

Cincinnati, OH 45202

(888) 793-WELL

A national organization of 21 centers providing emotional support, education, and hope for people with cancer. Offers a facilitated weekly online support group for women with breast cancer that meets on a secure chatroom requiring a code name for access. All services provided free of charge.

TREATMENT

Breast Cancer Treatment Guidelines for Patients (American Cancer Society and National Comprehensive Cancer Network, 2000), version 3. Go to www.nccn.org/patient_guidelines/breast_cancer/breast/Page1.htm or call ACS (800) ACS-2345 or NCCN (888) 909-NCCN.

Written by the National Comprehensive Cancer Network and the American Cancer Society. Patients will find treatment guidelines for breast cancer on this site. The guidelines examine types of breast cancer, staging, benign breast lumps, and diagnostic workup. Treatment, surgical procedures, and clinical trial information is also provided. Decision trees for each stage assist patients in evaluating treatment and follow-up options.

Note: Resources available in Spanish.

□ Colorado Health Net
www.coloradohealthnet.org/cancer/breast/treatment_toc.html
Breast Cancer Treatment Options discusses a variety of treatment options, with links to news articles on each specific treatment.

Enough Already! The Overtreatment of Early Breast Cancer, by George Goldberg (Paracelsus Press, 1996).
This brilliantly written book brings to the awareness of the general public the importance of patient-doctor dialogue, with respect to individual breast cancer diagnosis and medical treatment planning.

□ **National Cancer Institute:** *Understanding Breast Cancer Treatment*
http://rex.nci.nih.gov/PATIENTS/aboutbc/ubc_treatment.html
An online booklet entitled *Understanding Breast Cancer Treatment: A Guide for Patients* is provided on this site. This detailed guide examines the types of breast cancer, how it spreads, its causes, and gene testing. Staging, prognosis, and risk factors are also examined. Treatment options are explained, such as surgery, radiation therapy, and chemotherapy. Breast reconstruction as well as complementary therapies, emotional health, and follow-up care are also covered. A glossary and links for related resources are provided.

□ *Patients Guide to Breast Cancer.* Available at www.wehealnewyork. org or Beth Israel Medical Center, 10 Union Square East, New York, NY 10003, (212) 844-8468.
This pamphlet clarifies the complex terms and procedures surrounding diagnosis and treatment.
Note: Available in Spanish.

□ *A Patients Guide: Preventing and Treating Nausea and Vomiting Caused by Cancer Treatment* (American Society of Clinical Oncology, 2000). Call (888) 651-3038.

Twelve-page pamphlet contains guidelines for the use of antiemetic drugs to prevent and treat nausea and vomiting caused by cancer treatments.

□ *Understanding Breast Cancer Treatment* (P458, National Cancer Institute, 1998). Go to rex.nci.nih.gov or call (800) 4-CANCER.

This 72-page pamphlet contains lists of questions that will help a patient talk to her doctor about breast cancer. Topics covered include: early detection, diagnosis, treatment, adjuvant therapy, and reconstruction.

CHEMOTHERAPY AND RADIATION THERAPY

□ **CHEMOcare**
(800) 55-CHEMO or (908) 233-1103 in New Jersey
CHEMOcare is a nonprofit, voluntary program whose chief goal is to encourage people undergoing treatment for cancer to continue despite adverse side effects. Support is given by people who have survived a similar experience and have resumed living normal lives.

□ *Chemotherapy and You: A Guide to Self-Help during Treatment* (97-1136, 1999). Call (800) 4-CANCER.

A 56-page pamphlet, in question-and-answer format, addressing concerns of patients receiving chemotherapy. Emphasis is on explanation, self-help, and participation during treatment. Includes a glossary of terms.

The Chemotherapy Survival Guide, by Judith McKay, R.N., and Nancee Hirnao, R.N., M.S.N. (New Harbinger, 1993).

This book has material about coping with chemotherapy side effects like: nausea, fatigue, hair loss, skin changes, loss of appetite, and so on.

Coping with Chemotherapy: Authoritative Information and Compassionate Advice from a Chemotherapy Survivor, by Nancy Bruning (Avery/Penguin Putnam, 2002).

Bruning's candid and authoritative book fills the void of information available for patients facing this procedure. *Coping with Chemotherapy* is a must-read for anyone battling cancer.

□ *Helping Yourself during Chemotherapy: Four Steps for Patients* (94-3701, 1994). Call (800) 4-CANCER.

This easy-to-read 12-page brochure suggests four steps to follow during chemotherapy treatment.

Memorial Sloan-Kettering's Chemotherapy CD-ROM. Go to www.mskcc.org or Memorial Sloan-Kettering Cancer Center, 1275 York Avenue, New York, NY 10021, (212) 639-2000.

Developed by the medical experts at Memorial Sloan-Kettering Cancer Center, this CD-ROM teaches users how chemotherapy works and how to manage its side effects. Search under "Multimedia Patient Education" to print out a mail-in order form.

Radiation Oncology
http://oncolink.upenn.edu/specialty/rad_onc/
The University of Pennsylvania Cancer Centers Radiation Oncology from Oncolink links to various sites for radiation oncology.

□ *Radiation Therapy and You* (00-2227, 1998). Call (800) 4-CANCER.
This pamphlet was written for the patient receiving radiation therapy. It describes what to expect during therapy and offers helpful suggestions for self-care during and after treatment.

□ *Understanding Chemotherapy* (4458, 1998). Call (800) ACS-2345.
This pamphlet provides a brief introduction to chemotherapy, its benefits, and its side effects.

CLINICAL TRIALS

□ *Cancer Facts Questions and Answers: The Breast Cancer Prevention Trial* (1998). Call (800) 4-CANCER.
This fact sheet answers common questions about the Breast Cancer Prevention Trial, including its design, results, and significance for women. Free.

□ **Center Watch Clinical Trials Listing Services**
www.centerwatch.com
Includes more than 7,500 clinical trials that are actively recruiting patients.

☐ **NCI Clinical Trials**

http://cancertrials.nci.nih.gov

A comprehensive listing of all cancer clinical trials.

☐ **National Surgical Adjuvant Breast and Bowel Project**

www.nsabp.pitt.edu

3550 Terrace Street, Room 914

Pittsburgh, PA 15261

(412) 648-9720

The group responsible for most of the breast cancer clinical trials, including the tamoxifen prevention trial, STAR trial, and lumpectomy and radiation trial. Will let you know of physicians participating in their trials in your area.

☐ *Patient to Patient: Cancer Clinical Trials and You* (no. V112, National Institute of Health). Call (800) 4-CANCER.

Fifteen-minute videotape provides basic information regarding clinical trials.

☐ **PDQ (Physician Data Query)**

http://cancernet.nci.nih.gov (no "www" is necessary)

(800) 4-CANCER

The computerized cancer database of the NCI, providing information on treatment, organizations, doctors involved in cancer care, and a listing of more than 1,500 clinical trials that are open to patient accrual. Access by computer equipped with a modem and by fax.

☐ *Taking Part in Clinical Trials: What Cancer Patients Need to Know* (98-4250, 1998). Call (800) 4-CANCER.

Pamphlet for patients considering participating in cancer treatment trials; includes glossary.

Note: Resources available in Spanish.

LYMPHEDEMA

Breast Cancer Physical Therapy Center

1905 Spruce Street

Philadelphia, PA 19103

(215) 772-0160

Provides a pamphlet on exercises to help manage lymphedema. Cost is $8.95 (includes shipping/handling).

□ **Circle of Hope Lymphedema Foundation, Inc.**
www.lymphedemacircleofhope.org
36 Woodcrest Drive
Prospect, CT 06712
(203) 758-6138

This nonprofit corporation was developed to promote and provide educational programs, public awareness, medical treatment, and continued research for lymphedema.

Lymphedema: A Breast Cancer Patient's Guide to Prevention and Healing, by Jeannie Burt and Gwen White, P.T. (Hunter House, 1999).

This book talks about lymphedema, why it starts, and what can be done about it. It also includes stories of other women with lymphedema and shows what they are doing to manage and cope with their condition.

□ **The National Lymphedema Network and Network Hotline**
www.lymphnet.org
2211 Post Street, Suite 404
San Francisco, CA 94115
(800) 541-3259

This nonprofit organization provides patients and professionals with information about prevention and treatment of lymphedema. Call hotline for referrals for medical treatment, physical therapy, general information, and support in your area. They will send an information packet.

What Every Woman Facing Breast Cancer Should Know about Lymphedema: Hand and Arm Care Following Surgery or Radiation Therapy for Breast Cancer (0426, American Cancer Society, 2000). Call (800) ACS-2345.

This 16-page pamphlet explains lymphedema and offers basic guidelines for ways to help lower your risk of developing lymphedema or delaying its onset.

PAIN CONTROL

American Pain Foundation

www.painfoundation.org

(888) 615-PAIN (7246)

The American Pain Foundation is an independent, nonprofit organization serving people with pain, through information, education, and advocacy. Their mission is to improve the quality of life for people with pain by raising public awareness, providing practical information, promoting research, and advocating to remove barriers and increase access to effective pain management.

CancerFatigue.org

www.cancerfatigue.org

Fatigue is a problem for nearly all cancer patients, no matter the type of cancer or course of treatment. In an effort to improve patients' quality of life, this site from the Oncology Nursing Society explains what causes fatigue and offers practical advice for coping with it. Offers resources for both patients and caregivers. Email an oncology nurse your questions about treatment-related fatigue.

Note: Resources available in Spanish.

□ *Cancer Pain: Treatment Guidelines for Patients* (American Cancer Society and the National Comprehensive Cancer Network, 2001), version 1. Go to www.cancer.org or www.nccn.org or ACS (800) ACS-2345 or NCCN (888) 909-NCCN.

These guidelines were developed by a diverse panel of experts to provide clear and understandable information on cancer pain management; 31 pages.

Note: Resource available in Spanish.

□ **Managing Cancer Pain** (1994). Available from AHCPR Publications Clearinghouse, PO Box 8547, Silver Spring, MD 20907-8547, (800) 4-CANCER.

This consumer pamphlet details the guidelines of the U.S. government's Agency for Health Care Policy and Research for treating cancer pain.

☐ *Questions and Answers about Pain Control: A Guide for People with Cancer and Their Families* (4518-PS, 1995). Call (800) ACS-2345 or (800) 4-CANCER.

Discusses pain control using both medical and nonmedical methods; 76 pages.

SEEKING A SECOND OPINION

☐ *Clinical Practice Guidelines* (American Society of Clinical Oncology). www.asco.org/prof/pp/html/f_gs.htm.

Useful to use as a baseline for comparison with a doctor's recommendations. Doctors should be at least up to date on these.

☐ **R. A. Bloch Cancer Foundation, Inc.**

www.blochcancer.org

The R. A. Bloch Cancer Foundation matches newly diagnosed cancer patients with trained, home-based volunteers who have been treated for the same type of cancer. They also distribute informational materials, including a multidisciplinary list of institutions that offer second opinions.

Note: Resources available in Spanish.

TYPES OF BREAST CANCER/DISEASE

Diseases of the Breast, **edited by Jay Harris, M.D., Marc Lippman, M.D., Monica Morrow, M.D., and C. Kent Isborne, M.D.** (Lippincott, Williams, and Wilkins, 2000). To order, call (800) 877-2295 or go to www.lww.com.

Calcifications

☐ *Questions and Answers about Breast Calcifications* (95-3198, National Cancer Institute, 1997). Call (800) 4-CANCER.

This 3-page pamphlet discusses calcifications of the breast, their significance, and what can be done to treat them.

Ductal Carcinoma in Situ (DCIS)

Breastdoctor.com
www.breastdoctor.com/breast/cancer/DCIS.htm
Helpful place to embark on your DCIS research efforts.

Cancer BACUP
www.cancerbacup.org.uk/info/dcis.htm
Offers an explanation of DCIS diagnosis, treatment, and followup.

Oncolink, University of Pennsylvania Cancer Center
www.oncolink.upenn.edu/disease/breast/dcis/index.html
Ductal Carcinoma in Situ, A Guide for Patients is an introduction to DCIS.

Inflammatory Breast Cancer

☐ **Inflammatory Breast Cancer**
www.ibcsupport.org
Good information regarding the relatively rare inflammatory breast cancer.
Note: Information available in French, Spanish, Dutch, and Magaryul.

Male Breast Cancer

☐ **Adelphi Breast Cancer Support Program**
(800) 877-8077
Resources and a local support group for men with breast cancer.

☐ **Bridging the Gap Male Breast Cancer Awareness Group**
(503) 359-1483
Based in Portland, Oregon.

☐ **Male Breast Cancer**
http://interact.withus.com/interact/mbc
This site is for anyone dealing with male breast cancer, whether men
suffering from this disease, their doctors, other doctors interested in the disease, or researchers studying MBC. The site offers support groups, chat

rooms, discussion groups, and information about research, clinical trials, and treatment. To join, send an email message to: listserv@maelstrom. stjohns.edu. In the body of the message type: subscribe MaleBC [Your Name]. List owners: Bob Stafford, bstafford@skyenet.net; Steve Meredith, meredits@isomedia.com; and Gilles Frydman, gilles@dorsai.org.

☐ **Male Breast Cancer Telephone Support**
(262) 820-0856

☐ **The Susan G. Komen Breast Cancer Foundation**
www.breastcancerinfo.com/bhealth/html/male_breast_cancer.asp
(800) IM-AWARE
This website answers common questions concerning male breast cancer.

INTERNATIONAL RESOURCES

Action Cancer: Belfast, Ireland
http://hostcd.aware.easynet.co.uk/index.htm
A local charity in Ireland, committed to fighting breast and cervical cancer since 1978, Action Cancer has a full-time clinic and mobile unit for early detection screening and provides one-to-one counseling. Services are free of charge. Action Cancer also funds a leading research team at Queen's University.

The Association of European Cancer Leagues (ECL)
http://ecl.uicc.org/
A nonprofit, nonpolitical, and nonsectarian association whose aim is to promote health; reduce the risk of disease; promote research and evidence-based treatment in the field of cancer; and to be responsive to the needs of cancer patients, their families, and caregivers.

The Australian Cancer Society
www.cancer.org.au
70 William Street
East Sydney NSW 2010

Australia

02 9380 9022

An Australian organization similar to the American Cancer Society.

Australian New Zealand Breast Cancer Trials Group
Department of Clinical Oncology
Newcastle Mater Hospital
Waratah NSW 2298
Australia
+61 2 4921 1155

A group dedicated to the research of breast cancer in Australia and New Zealand. Contact them for more information on the latest clinical trials being conducted.

Breast Cancer Action Nova Scotia
www.bcans.org

A survivor-driven group, online since 1996, providing consistent support services to the global community. Site houses over 70,000 archived and current messages and receives over 1,000 visitors a day. With over 200 survivor stories and multiple discussion forums, BCANS has developed an active breast cancer online community.

Breast Cancer Care: London, England
www.breastcancercare.org.uk/splash

A national organization offering information and support to women and men with breast cancer, and their partners, families, and friends. Services are free, confidential, and accessible, and include: a national helpline, information, volunteer services, aftercare services, and regional services. It also provides information to the general public, health professionals, and the media.

Breast Cancer Society of Canada
www.bcsc.ca/

Targets women's health issues. Funds research into the detection, treatment, and prevention of breast cancer and promotes public awareness.

British Complementary Medicine Association (BCMA)
www.bcma.co.uk
PO Box 2074

Seaford BN25 1HQ
England
0845 345 5977
This umbrella organization produces a guide and a code of conduct for practitioners and holds a register of practitioners.

British Holistic Medical Association
www.bhma.org
59 Lansdowne Place
Hove
East Sussex BN3 1FL
England
01273 725951
Provides information, produces self-help tapes, booklets, and a quarterly magazine.

British Medical Acupuncture Society
www.medical-acupuncture.co.uk
12 Marbury House
Higher Whitley
Warrington
Cheshire WA4 4QW
England
01925 730727
Information service and provides a list of members.

Brustkrebs-Initiative, Hilfe zur Brusthgesundheit
www.brustkrebs.net
A German-language breast cancer activism site.

Canadian Breast Cancer Foundation
790 Bay Street, Suite 1000
Toronto, Ontario M5G 1N8
Canada
(800) 387-9816 or (416) 596-6773
This organization offers financial support for research and treatment of breast cancer and encourages and coordinates training, public information, and all related resources.

Canadian/French Language Sources
www.cbcn.ca

Canadian Breast Cancer Network is a survivor-directed, national network of organizations and individuals. There are both links to Canadian resources and groups and links to French-language sites on breast cancer.

CancerBACUP
www.cancerbacup.org.uk
3 Bath Place, Rivington Street
London EC2A 3JR
England
0808 800 1234, or 020 7613 2121

CancerBACUP aims to help people live with cancer by providing information, emotional support, and counseling for patients, their families, and health care professionals. It is recognized as the foremost provider of cancer information in the United Kingdom. The CancerBACUP website features fact sheets on different types of cancers and individual chemotherapy and hormonal therapy drugs.

Cancer Information Services of the Canadian Cancer Society
www.cancer.ca
(888) 939-3333 for calls from Canada only
Note: Information service in English and French.

Council for Complementary and Alternative Medicine (CCAM)
63 Jeddo Road
London W12 6HQ
England
020 8735 0632

An umbrella organization for the main CAM therapies.

Europa Donna: Europe
http://hosted.aware.easynet.co.uk/contacts/europa

Europa Donna is the European breast cancer coalition, which currently involves membership from 19 countries. The goals of the organization are to increase public awareness of the issues concerning breast cancer, to encourage breast cancer research, and to support the breast cancer patient. Each country welcomes membership to its Europa Donna National Forum, which undertakes a variety of activities in support of its priority goals. International exchange of information and experience is encouraged between member countries. A newsletter is published and an international conference is held biannually.

The European Organization for Research and Treatment of Cancer (EORTC)

www.eortc.be

Maintains information about clinical trials being conducted in European countries.

Gilda's Club Montreal, Inc.

www.gildasclub.org

(514) 937-3636

Gilda's Club, a free, nonprofit program, provides social and emotional support to cancer patients, their families, and friends. Lectures, workshops, networking groups, special events, and a children's program are available.

International Cancer Information Services

http://cis.nci.nih.gov/resources/intlist.htm

Offers services similar to those the United States Cancer Information Service offers to their own citizens, as well as to American citizens living outside the United States. A more comprehensive list of international cancer organizations is available through the International Union Against Cancer.

The International Cancer Information Service Group (ICISG)

http://icisg.uicc.org/index.htm

The International Cancer Information Service Group is a network of world Cancer Information Services working under the auspices of the International Union Cancer Control (UICC) and provides information and resources on all aspects of cancer for those people concerned or affected by cancer.

The International Union Against Cancer (UICC)

www.uicc.org

The International Union Against Cancer consists of international cancer-related organizations devoted to the worldwide fight against cancer. These organizations serve as resources for the public and may have helpful information about cancer, treatment centers, and research studies. The UICC maintains a list of its *member* organizations as well as a *directory* of cancer-concerned organizations around the world.

iSource National Breast Cancer Centre (The Centre)

www.nbcc.org.au
PO Box 572, Kings Cross
Sydney NSW 1340
Australia
(02) 9334 1700, +61-2-9326-9329 (international)

The iSource National Breast Cancer Centre (The Centre) was established in March 1995 by the Commonwealth government in response to community concerns about the human costs of breast cancer. The Centre can provide women with an up-to-date list of Australian and international resources available to women about breast cancer, including pamphlets, books, tapes, and so on. Copies of or contact points for many of these resources are available by mail or through its resource center in Sydney, a local contact point, or the NBCC coordinator based in each state or territory cancer organization.

The Scottish Breast Cancer Campaign: Edinburgh, Scotland

www.scottishbreastcancercampaign.org

The Scottish Breast Cancer Campaign (a nonparty political pressure group made up of breast cancer patients and their families and friends) strives for *all* women throughout Scotland to receive the best possible treatment, to be aware of breast cancer and their rights as patients, and for increased funding (equally shared throughout Scotland) for treatment, staffing, and research.

Glossary

A33 monoclonal antibody: A type of monoclonal antibody used in cancer detection or therapy. Monoclonal antibodies are laboratory-produced substances that can locate and bind to cancer cells.

Acini: The parts of the breast gland where fluid or milk is produced.

Adenocarcinoma: A form of cancer that involves cells from the lining of the walls of many different organs of the body. Breast cancer is a type of adenocarcinoma.

Adenoma: A noncancerous tumor.

Adjuvant therapies: Treatments (e.g., chemotherapy, radiation therapy, and/or hormonal therapy) given in addition to a primary therapy to increase the chances of successful treatment of the disease or decrease the chances of recurrence. Adjuvant therapies are often scheduled soon after surgery.

Advanced breast cancer: Breast cancer that has spread from the primary site to other sites in the body.

Aggressive: A quickly growing cancer.

Alopecia: The medical name for hair loss. This is a common side effect of chemotherapy, since it interferes with fast-growing cells, including those that produce hair.

Alternative therapies: Practices that have not been proven to the clinical standards of modern Western medicine. Alternative medicine includes such practices as dietary supplements, megadose vitamins, herbal preparations, special teas, massage therapy, magnet therapy, spiritual healing, and meditation.

Amenorrhea: The absence or discontinuation of menstrual periods.

Analgesics: Drugs that reduce pain. These drugs include aspirin, acetaminophen, and ibuprofen.

Anaplastic: A term used to describe cancer cells that divide rapidly and bear little or no resemblance to normal cells.

Androgen: A male sex hormone used to treat recurring breast cancer by blocking the activity of estrogen, a female hormone that fuels the growth of some breast cancers.

Anemia: A condition in which the number of red blood cells is below normal.

Anesthesia: Loss of feeling or awareness. Local anesthetics cause loss of feeling in a part of the body. General anesthetics put a person to sleep.

Aneuploid: The characteristic of having either fewer or more than the normal number of chromosomes in a cell. This is an abnormal cell.

Angiogenesis: Blood vessel formation. Tumor angiogenesis is the growth of blood vessels from surrounding tissue into a solid tumor. This is caused by the release of a chemical by the tumor cells.

Antibiotics: Drugs used to treat infection.

Antibodies: Proteins produced by certain white blood cells in response to foreign substances (antigens). Each antibody can bind only to a specific antigen. The purpose of this binding is to help destroy the antigen.

Antiemetic: A medicine that prevents or relieves nausea and vomiting used during and sometimes after chemotherapy.

Antiestrogen: A class of drugs that bind with estrogen receptors to prevent tumor growth in cases of hormonally sensitive cancer. Tamoxifen is an example of this type of drug.

Antigens: Substances that are recognized by the immune system and cause the immune system to create antibodies.

Apoptosis: A normal series of events in a cell that lead to its death.

Areola: The area of dark-colored skin on the breast that surrounds the nipple.

Aromatase inhibitors: These drugs work by binding to the body's aromatase enzyme, an enzyme responsible for producing estrogen. Many breast cancer cells depend on estrogen to grow and multiply quickly. Once the aromatase inhibitor has binded to the aromatase enzyme, estrogen cannot be produced by the enzyme. This lack of estrogen starves cancer cells, preventing them from growing and dividing.

Aspiration: Removing fluid or cells from tissue by inserting a needle into an area and drawing the fluid into the syringe.

Asymptomatic: Without obvious signs or symptoms of disease. Cancer may cause symptoms and warning signs, but especially in its early stages, cancer may develop and grow without producing any symptoms.

Atypical cells: Not usual; abnormal. Cancer is the result of atypical cell division.

Atypical ductal hyperplasia (ADH): Abnormal growth of tissue cells in the milk duct of the breast.

Atypical hyperplasia: Tissue cells that display abnormal characteristics and are often considered precancerous.

Atypical lobular hyperplasia (ALH): Abnormal growth of tissue cells in the lobule of the breast.

Autologous bone marrow transplant: A complex procedure used to treat advanced or recurring breast cancer. A portion of the bone marrow is removed from the cancer patient and cleansed, treated, and stored. The patient is treated with either high doses of chemotherapy or radiation therapy, which destroy the cancer cells and the remaining bone marrow. The stored bone marrow is then transplanted back into the patient.

Axilla: The underarm or armpit.

Axillary lymph node dissection: Surgery to remove lymph nodes found in the armpit region.

Axillary lymph nodes: Lymph nodes located in the underarm area. The axillary lymph nodes are categorized as level I, level II, or level III, on the basis of their location relative to the pectoralis minor muscle.

Benign: Not cancerous; does not invade nearby tissue or spread to other parts of the body.

Bilateral breast cancer: Cases in which breast cancer can be found in both breasts. In nearly all instances of bilateral breast cancer, there are two separate breast cancers (one in each breast), rather than spread of the same breast cancer from one side to the other.

Bilateral mastectomy: Surgical removal of all or parts of both breasts.

Biomarkers: Substances sometimes found in an increased amount in the blood, other body fluids, or tissues and that may suggest the presence of some types of cancer.

Biopsy specimen: Tissue removed from the body and examined under a microscope to determine if disease is present.

Blood count: A test to measure the number of red blood cells (RBCs), white blood cells (WBCs), and platelets in a blood sample.

Blood transfusion: The administration of blood or blood products into a blood vessel.

Bone marrow: The soft, spongelike tissue in the center of large bones that produces white blood cells, red blood cells, and platelets.

Bone metastases: Cancer that has spread from the original (primary) tumor to the bone.

Brachytherapy: Radioactive material sealed in needles, seeds, wires, or catheters is placed directly into or near the tumor. Also called internal radiation therapy or implant radiation.

Brain metastases: Cancer that has spread from the original (primary) tumor to the brain.

BRCA1: A gene located on chromosome 17 that normally helps to suppress cell growth. Inheriting an altered version of BRCA1 predisposes an individual to breast cancer.

BRCA2: A gene located on chromosome 13. Inheriting an altered version of BRCA1 predisposes an individual to breast cancer.

Breast cancer: Abnormal cells that originate in the breast and grow and divide out of control, creating a mass of tissue (tumor) in the breast. Breast cancer originates in the breast tissue, but like other cancers, it can invade and grow into the tissue surrounding the breast and travel to other parts of the body and form new tumors.

Breast conservation surgery: Breast surgery aimed at sparing the majority of breast tissue so that, when fully clothed, there is the appearance of a normal breast. The surgical procedures used in breast conservation include lumpectomy, segmental mastectomy, and quadrantectomy. Lumpectomy is the least disfiguring of the breast conservation procedures. Breast conservation surgery is usually combined with radiation therapy to decrease the chances of breast cancer recurrence.

Breast implant: A round or teardrop-shaped sac inserted into the body to restore the shape of the breast following a mastectomy. May be filled with saline water or synthetic material.

Breast prosthesis: A breast-shaped form, for placement within a bra or bathing suit, to provide the appearance of an intact breast following a mastectomy. Breast prostheses are available in a variety of shapes, sizes, and colors.

Breast reconstruction: Surgery to rebuild a breast's shape after a mastectomy. The surgery is usually performed by a plastic surgeon. Breast reconstruction can begin at the time of mastectomy (immediate reconstruction) or at a point in time after the mastectomy has been performed. The success of a breast reconstruction procedure can be affected by treatments received for breast cancer, individual body characteristics, and personal lifestyle habits.

Breast self-examination (BSE): One of three tests the American Cancer Society recommends to help detect breast cancer in its earliest stages. The goal of these early detection tests is to find cancers early enough to give women the best chance of living a long life. By regularly examining her own breasts, a woman is likely to notice any changes that occur.

CA-125: Substance sometimes found in an increased amount in the blood, other body fluids, or tissues and that may suggest the presence of some types of cancer.

Calcifications: Small calcium deposits in breast tissue. They are the smallest object detected on mammography.

Cancer: A general term used to describe more than 100 different uncontrolled growths of abnormal cells in the body. Cancer cells have the ability to continue to grow, invade, and destroy surrounding tissue, leave the original site, and travel via lymph or blood systems to other parts of the body where they can set up new cancerous tumors.

Cancer of unknown primary origin: Cancer cells are found in the body, but the place where the cells first started growing (the origin or primary site) cannot be found.

Carcinogen: Any substance that initiates or promotes the development of cancer.

Carcinoma: A form of cancer that develops in tissues covering or lining organs of the body, such as the skin, the uterus, the lung, or the breast.

Carcinoma in situ: An early stage of development, when the cancer is still confined to the tissues of origin. It has not spread outside the area. In situ carcinomas are highly curable.

Cathepsin D: An enzyme released by breast cancer cells.

CAT scan or CT scan: An X-ray view of the body in sections. Also called computerized tomography scans.

Catheter: A flexible tube used to deliver fluids into or withdraw fluids from the body.

Cell: The basic structural unit of all life. All living matter is composed of cells.

Cell proliferation: An increase in the number of cells as a result of cell growth and cell division.

Centimeter: A unit of measure. One centimeter (abbreviated as "cm") equals 0.4 inches. There are approximately 2.5 centimeters to 1 inch.

c-erbB-2: The gene that controls cell growth by making the human epidermal growth factor receptor 2. Also called HER2/neu.

Chemoprevention: The use of drugs, vitamins, or other agents to try to reduce the risk of or delay the development or recurrence of cancer. In the case of breast cancer, it is tamoxifen or SERMs (selective estrogen receptor modulators).

Chemosensitivity assay: A laboratory test to analyze the responsiveness of a tumor to a specific drug.

Chemotherapy: Treatment of cancer by use of chemicals. Usually refers to drugs used to treat cancer.

Chromosome: Part of a cell that contains genetic information. Except for sperm and eggs, all human cells contain 46 chromosomes.

Chronic: A disease or condition that persists or progresses over a long period of time.

Clinical exam: A physical examination in which the doctor relies on visual inspection and touch.

Clinical staging: A determination of the extent of cancer progression that is based on the results of clinical exam, imaging methods such as mammography, and pathological examination of tissue removed from the breast and/or other sites during biopsy.

Clinical trial: Medical research study designed to test the safety and/or effectiveness of new medications or procedures. Individuals participating in clinical trials must be made aware of the possible risks and benefits of trial participation and provide their informed consent.

Combination chemotherapy: Treatment with multiple chemotherapy drugs.

Combined modality therapy: Cancer treatment involving more than one type of therapeutic approach or "modality." An example is the use of radiation therapy, hormonal therapy, and chemotherapy in the same breast cancer patient.

Complementary therapies: Therapies that have not been scientifically tested and approved by regulatory agencies (such as the FDA) that may be used alongside conventional Western medicine.

Complete blood count (CBC): A laboratory test to determine the number of red blood cells, white blood cells, platelets, hemoglobin, and other components of a blood sample.

Compression bandage: A bandage designed to provide pressure to a particular area.

Consolidation therapy: Chemotherapy treatments given after induction chemotherapy to further reduce the number of cancer cells.

Contralateral: Located on the opposite side of the body.

Cooper's ligaments: Flexible bands of tissue that pass from the chest muscle between the lobes of the breasts, providing shape and support to the breasts.

Core needle aspiration biopsy (also known as core-cutting needle biopsy; see also **needle biopsy**): Removal of breast tissue samples using a large-diameter needle. The samples are examined by a pathologist, who determines whether they are benign or malignant.

Cyst: An abnormal saclike structure that contains liquid or semisolid material. Usually benign. Lumps in the breast are often found to be harmless cysts.

Cytology: Study of cells under a microscope that have been sloughed off, cut out of, or scraped off organs to microscopically examine for signs of cancer.

Definitive treatment: Treatment aimed at curing disease rather than controlling symptoms.

DES (diethylstilbestrol): A synthetic hormone that was prescribed from the early 1940s until 1971 to help women with complications of pregnancy, DES has been linked to an increased risk of clear cell carcinoma of the vagina in daughters of women who had used DES. May also increase the risk of breast cancer in women who used DES.

Detection: The discovery of an abnormality in an asymptomatic or symptomatic person.

Diagnosis: The process of identifying a disease by its characteristic signs, symptoms, and laboratory findings. With cancer, the earlier the diagnosis is made, the better the chance for successful treatment.

Diagnostic mammogram: Mammogram or ultrasound performed to investigate a palpable lump or a suspicious site detected on a routine screening mammogram.

Differentiated: The similarity between a normal cell and the cancer cell; defines what degree of change has occurred. Cancer cells that are well differentiated are close to the original cell and are usually less aggressive. Poorly differentiated cells have changed more and are more aggressive.

Diploid: The characteristic of having two sets of chromosomes in a cell. This is normal for a breast cell.

Disclosure laws: Laws requiring physicians to present all treatment options to patients before initiating a treatment.

Disease progression: Cancer that continues to grow or spread.

DNA: One of two nucleic acids (the other is RNA) found in the nucleus of all cells. Contains genetic information on cell growth, division, and cell function.

Dose-intensive chemotherapy: A chemotherapy regimen in which the drugs are administered at their standard doses but within a shorter time interval than usual.

Dose rate: The strength of a treatment given over a period of time.

Doubling time: The time required for a cell to double in number. Breast cancer has been shown to double in size every 23 to 209 days. It would take one cell, doubling every 100 days, 8 to 10 years to reach 1 centimeter or ⅜ inch.

Ductal carcinoma in situ (DCIS): Abnormal cells that involve only the lining of a duct. The cells have not spread outside the duct to other tissues in the breast. Also called intraductal carcinoma.

Ductal papillomas: Small noncancerous fingerlike growths in the mammary duct that may cause a bloody nipple discharge. Commonly found in women 45 to 50 years of age.

Ducts: Tubelike structures in the breast. In women who are breast-feeding, milk is transported through these ducts on its way toward the nipple. Ductal carcinomas (whether in situ or invasive) originate from the cells lining the inner surface of the ducts.

Dysplasia: Cells that look abnormal under a microscope but are not necessarily cancer.

Early-stage breast cancer (or early breast cancer): Breast cancer classified as stage I or stage II with a primary tumor that is no larger than 5 centimeters (about 2 inches) in size.

Edema: Swelling caused by fluid accumulation in a particular area of the body.

Encapsulated: Confined to a specific, localized area and surrounded by a thin layer of tissue.

Erythrocytes: Cells that carry oxygen to all parts of the body. Also called red blood cells (RBCs).

Estrogen: A female hormone produced by the ovaries, adrenal glands, and fatty tissues. Estrogen regulates menstruation, reproduction, and the growth of secondary sex characteristics (e.g., breasts). It may also activate some forms of breast cancer.

Estrogen receptor: A protein in breast cancer and other cells to which estrogen attaches. The presence of a large number of estrogen receptors on breast cancer cells indicates that estrogen contributes to the growth of the cancer. The presence of a small or negligible number of estrogen receptors indicates that the growth of the cancer is not influenced by the presence of estrogen.

Estrogen receptor status: Determination of whether a tumor's cells contain large or small numbers of estrogen receptors. If the estrogen receptor status is *positive,* the cells contain large numbers of receptors, and there is a good chance that hormonal therapies such as tamoxifen will be effective. If the estrogen receptor status is *negative,* the cells contain small numbers of receptors, and there is less likelihood that hormonal therapies will be effective.

Estrogen replacement therapy: Estrogen treatment for women who have already undergone menopause.

Etiology: The cause or origin of disease.

Excisional biopsy: A surgical procedure in which an entire lump or suspicious area is removed for diagnosis. The tissue is then examined under a microscope.

External-beam radiation: Radiation therapy that uses a machine to aim high-energy rays at the cancer. Also called external radiation.

Fat necrosis tumor: Destruction of fat cells in the breast because of trauma or injury, can cause a hard noncancerous lump.

Fibroadenoma: A noncancerous, solid tumor most commonly found in younger women.

Fibrocystic breast changes or condition: A noncancerous breast condition in which multiple cysts or lumpy areas develop in one or both breasts. It can be accompanied by discomfort or pain that fluctuates with the menstrual cycle. Large cysts can be treated by aspiration of the fluid they contain.

Fine needle aspiration (FNA) biopsy: A procedure in which a thin needle is inserted to remove, for microscopic evaluation, fluid from a cyst or cells from a tumor. Also called needle biopsy.

Free flap: Breast reconstruction method that uses muscle, skin, and fat that is removed from another area of the body.

Frozen section: A technique in which a part of the biopsy tissue is frozen immediately, and a thin slice is then mounted on a microscope slide, enabling a pathologist to analyze it in just a few minutes for a diagnosis. Pathologists do not recommend doing a frozen section on breast tissue, since fatty tissue freezes poorly and can give a false positive or false negative result.

Gamma knife: Radiation therapy in which high-energy rays are aimed at a tumor from many angles in a single treatment session.

Gene: The functional and physical unit of heredity passed from parent to offspring. Genes are pieces of DNA, and most genes contain the information for making a specific protein.

Genetic: Inherited; having to do with information that is passed from parents to children through genes in sperm and egg cells.

Genetic markers: Alterations in DNA that may indicate an increased risk of developing a specific disease or disorder.

Genetic testing: Analyzing DNA to look for a genetic alteration that may indicate an increased risk for developing a specific disease or disorder.

Grading: A system for classifying cancer cells in terms of how abnormal they appear when examined under a microscope. The objective of a grading system is to provide information about the probable growth rate of the tumor and its tendency to spread. The systems used to grade tumors vary with each type of cancer. Grading plays a role in treatment decisions.

Guidance method: An imaging procedure for locating suspicious sites in the breast that can be detected by mammography or ultrasound but not by touch (i.e., no lump can be felt). Guidance methods are used for performing fine needle aspiration and core needle biopsies and for performing wire or needle localization in preparation for excisional biopsy or lumpectomy. In some cases, computerized tomography (CAT scan) is the imaging procedure that is used.

Guidelines: A series of recommendations developed by an organization or government agency for screening, diagnosis, or treatment.

Halsted radical mastectomy: See **total radical mastectomy.**

Hematoma: A collection of blood that can form in a wound after surgery, after an aspiration, or from an injury.

High-dose chemotherapy: Administration of chemotherapy drugs at high doses. The goal of high-dose chemotherapy is to kill more tumor cells than is possible with chemotherapy drugs at conventional doses.

Histopathologic type of breast cancer: The classification of breast cancer type based on its microscopic appearance.

Histopathology: The study of disease via the microscopic examination of tissue.

Hormonal therapy: Treatment of cancer by removing, blocking, or adding hormones. Also called endocrine therapy. The drugs used are SERMs (selective estrogen receptor modulators).

Hormone receptor test: A test to measure the amount of certain proteins, called hormone receptors, in cancer tissue. Hormones can attach to these proteins. A high level of hormone receptors may mean that hormones help the cancer grow.

Hormone receptor status: Determination of whether a tumor's cells contain large or small numbers of *estrogen* and *progesterone* receptors.

Hormone replacement therapy (HRT): Hormones (estrogen and/or progesterone) given to postmenopausal women or women who have had their ovaries surgically removed in order to replace the estrogen no longer produced by the ovaries.

Hormones: Chemicals produced by glands in the body and circulated in the bloodstream. Hormones control the actions of certain cells or organs.

Human epidermal growth factor receptor 2: A protein found on the surface of some breast cancer cells that allows epidermal growth factor to stimulate cell growth. Also called HER2/neu or c-erbB-2.

Hyperplasia: An abnormal increase in the number of cells in an organ or tissue.

Imagery: A technique in which the person focuses on positive images in the mind.

Imaging: Tests that produce pictures of areas inside the body.

Immune adjuvant: A drug that stimulates the immune system to respond to disease.

Immune response: The activity of the immune system against foreign substances (antigens).

Immune system: Complex system by which the body protects itself from outside invaders, which are harmful to the body.

Immunodeficiency: The decreased ability of the body to fight infection and disease.

Immunosuppression: Suppression of the body's immune system and its ability to fight infections or disease. Immunosuppression may be deliberately induced with drugs, as in preparation for bone marrow or other organ transplantation, in order to prevent rejection of the donor tissue.

Immunotherapy: Treatment to stimulate or restore the ability of the person's immune system to fight infection and disease. Also used to reduce side effects that may be caused by some cancer treatments. Also called biological therapy or biological response modifier (BRM) therapy.

Incidence: The number of new cases of a disease diagnosed each year.

Incision: A cut made in the body during surgery.

Incisional biopsy: Surgical procedure to remove, for microscopic evaluation, a portion of a suspicious site or tumor.

Infiltrating cancer: Cancer that has spread beyond the layer of tissue in which it developed and is growing into surrounding, healthy tissues. Also called invasive cancer.

Inflammation: Reaction of tissue to various conditions, which may result in pain, redness, or warmth of tissues in the area.

Inflammatory breast cancer: A type of breast cancer in which the breast looks red or has the presence of a rash, and/or is swollen, and feels warm. The skin of the breast may also show the pitted appearance called peau d'orange (like the skin of an orange). The redness and warmth occur because the cancer cells block the lymph vessels in the skin.

Informed consent: Permission granted by an individual or an individual's legal representative to perform a procedure or treatment after risks and possible complications have been explained.

Infusion: The introduction of a fluid, including drugs, into the bloodstream. Also called intravenous infusion.

In situ: "In place"; localized and confined to one area. A very early stage of cancer.

Internal radiation: Radiation therapy that is given internally. This is done by placing radioactive material that is sealed in needles, seeds, wires, or catheters directly into or near the tumor. Also called implant radiation or brachytherapy.

Intraductal carcinoma: Abnormal cells that involve only the lining of a duct. The cells have not spread outside the duct to other tissues in the breast. Also called ductal carcinoma in situ (DCIS); the very earliest stage of breast cancer—stage 0. Also called non-invasive breast cancer.

Intraoperative radiation therapy (IORT): Radiation treatment aimed directly at a tumor during surgery.

Intravenous (IV): Injected into a blood vessel.

Invasive cancer: Cancer that has spread beyond the layer of tissue in which it developed and is growing into surrounding, healthy tissues. Also called infiltrating cancer.

Inverted nipple: The turning inward of the nipple. Usually a congenital condition, but if it occurs where it has not previously existed, it can be a sign of breast cancer.

Investigational drug: A medication being studied in clinical trials to determine if it is safe and effective for treating a particular condition. A drug ceases to be investigational when the U.S. Food and Drug Administration has approved it for the specific purpose for which it is being proposed.

Ipsilateral: Located on the same side of the body.

Keloid: A thick, irregular scar caused by excessive tissue growth at the site of an incision or wound.

Killer cells: White blood cells that attack tumor cells and body cells that have been invaded by foreign substances.

Lactation: Process of producing milk from the breasts.

Laser: A device that concentrates light into an intense, narrow beam used to cut or destroy tissue. It is used in microsurgery, photodynamic therapy, and for a variety of diagnostic purposes.

Latissimus dorsi flap: Method for breast reconstruction in which the muscle from the upper part of the back is used to form a structure that resembles the breast that was removed during mastectomy.

Lesion: An abnormal tissue mass or tumor.

Linear accelerator: A machine that produces high-energy X-ray beams to destroy cancer cells.

Lobe: A portion of an organ such as the liver, lung, breast, or brain.

Lobular carcinoma in situ (LCIS): Abnormal cells found in the lobules of the breast. This condition seldom becomes invasive cancer. However, having lobular carcinoma in situ increases one's risk of developing breast cancer in either breast and is considered a marker for being high risk.

Lobular neoplasia: See **lobular carcinoma in situ.**

Localized: Restricted to the site of origin without evidence of spread.

Localized cancer: A cancer still confined to its site of origin.

Local recurrence: Recurrence of cancer in the breast after lumpectomy or in scar tissue or remaining breast tissue after mastectomy.

Local therapy: Treatment that affects cells in the tumor and the area close to it.

Lump: Any kind of abnormal mass in the breast or elsewhere in the body.

Lumpectomy: The surgical removal of a tumor and some of the surrounding normal tissue. The goal of lumpectomy is to preserve as much of the breast as possible, so that there is the appearance of a normal intact breast. Also known as breast conservation surgery.

Lymph: A clear fluid circulating throughout the body in the lymphatic system that contains white blood cells and antibodies.

Lymphatic system: The system of channels through which lymph moves in the body.

Lymphatic vessels: Vessels that remove cellular waste from the body by filtering through lymph nodes and eventually emptying into the vascular (blood) system.

Lymphedema: A condition in which excess lymph collects in tissue and causes swelling. It may occur in the arm or leg after lymph vessels or lymph nodes in the underarm or groin are removed.

Lymph node drainage: The flow of lymph from an area of tissue into a particular lymph node.

Lymph node mapping: The use of dyes and radioactive substances to identify lymph nodes that contain tumor cells. See **sentinel lymph node**.

Lymph nodes: Small organs located throughout the body along the channels of the lymphatic system. The lymph nodes store special cells that fight infection and other diseases. Clusters of lymph nodes are found in the underarms, groin, neck, chest, and abdomen. Also called lymph glands.

Magnetic resonance imaging (MRI): A magnet scan; a form of X ray using magnets instead of radiation. Gives a more clearly defined picture of fatty tissue than X ray.

Magnification view: Special enlarged views to magnify an area for greater detail of abnormal or suspicious finding. Used in mammography.

Malignant tumor: A mass of cancer cells. These cells have uncontrolled growth and will invade surrounding tissues and spread to distant sites of the body, setting up new cancer sites, a process called metastasis.

Mammary duct ectasia: A noncancerous breast disease most often found in women during menopause. The ducts in or beneath the nipple become clogged with cellular and fatty debris. The duct may have gray to greenish discharge and a lump you can feel and that can become inflamed, causing pain.

Mammary glands: The breast glands that produce and carry milk by way of the mammary ducts to the nipples during pregnancy and breast-feeding.

Mammogram (see also **diagnostic mammogram** and **screening mammogram**): An X ray of the breast used to assess a lump, or as preventive screening in individuals who show no signs of breast cancer during clinical exam.

Mammotest: Biopsy (stereotactic) performed under mammography while breast is compressed and lump is viewed by physician. Sample of lump is removed, using a large core needle, and is sent to lab to determine if it is benign or malignant.

Margins: The area of tissue surrounding a tumor when it is removed by surgery.

Mastalgia: Pain occurring in the breast.

Mastectomy: Surgical procedure to remove an entire breast, nipple, areola, and possibly some surrounding tissue for the treatment or prevention of breast cancer. In some cases, where mastectomy is immediately followed by reconstructive surgery, the nipple is kept intact.

Modified radical mastectomy: The most common type of mastectomy. Breast, skin, nipple, areola, and underarm lymph nodes are removed. The chest muscles are preserved intact.

Prophylactic mastectomy: A procedure sometimes recommended for patients at a very high risk for developing cancer in one or both breasts.

Subcutaneous mastectomy: Performed before cancer is detected, removes the breast tissue but leaves the outer skin, areola, and nipple intact. *Subcutanous Mastectomy is not considered an appropriate treatment for invasive or noninvasive breast cancer.*

Total radical mastectomy (Halsted radical): The surgical removal of the breast, breast skin, nipple, areola, chest muscles, and underarm lymph nodes.

Segmental mastectomy (partial mastectomy/lumpectomy): A surgical procedure in which only a portion of the breast is removed, including the cancer and the surrounding margin of healthy breast tissue.

Total simple mastectomy: Surgical removal of entire breast, without co-removal of the underlying chest muscles or axillary lymph nodes.

Mastitis: Infection occurring in the breast. Pain, tenderness, swelling, redness, and warmth may be observed. Usually related to infection and will respond to antibiotic treatment.

Medial: Located centrally or toward the center of the body.

Medical oncologist: A physician who specializes in treating cancer primarily through chemotherapy and hormonal therapy.

Metastasis: The spread of cancer from the primary tumor to other parts of the body. The most common sites for breast metastasis are lung, bone, and liver.

Microcalcifications: Tiny deposits of calcium in the breast that cannot be felt but can be detected on a mammogram. A cluster of these very small specks of calcium may indicate that cancer is present.

Microcyst: A cyst that is too small to be felt but may be observed on mammography or ultrasound screening.

Micrometastasis: Undetectable spread of cancer outside of the breast that is not seen on routine screening tests. Metastasis is too limited to have created enough mass to be detected easily—may be discovered by cytology.

Multicentric: When multiple tumors are detected in different regions of the same anatomical structure. For breast cancer, multicentric tumors are located in different "quadrants" of the same breast or, according to some professionals, at distances greater than 5 centimeters (about 2 inches) within the same breast.

Mutation: A permanent change in the genetic code of DNA that can be caused by exposure to chemicals or ultraviolet light or to mistakes that occur during DNA replication. Mutations can lead to cancer or to birth defects.

Necrosis: Death of a tissue.

Needle biopsy: The removal of tissue or fluid with a needle for examination under a microscope. Also called a fine needle aspiration.

Needle localization: A procedure used to "mark" the boundaries of suspicious sites within the breast. Thin needles are used in preparation for removal by a surgeon during excisional biopsy or lumpectomy. Ultrasound or stereotactic is usually used to identify the sites that need to be marked.

Negative axillary lymph nodes: Lymph nodes in the armpit that show no evidence of cancer.

Neoadjuvant chemotherapy: Treatment with drugs to destroy cancer cells and shrink the tumor before it is removed by surgery.

Neoadjuvant therapy: Treatment given before the primary treatment. Neoadjuvant therapy can be chemotherapy, radiation therapy, or hormone therapy.

Neoplasm: Any abnormal growth. Neoplasms may be benign or malignant, but the term usually is used to describe a cancer.

Nipple discharge: Any fluid, other than milk in breast-feeding mothers, that leaks or can be squeezed from the nipple. This fluid can be clear, milky, bloody, tan, gray, or green.

Nipple discharge smear: A thin layer of nipple fluid spread on a slide for microscopic examination.

Node-negative: Cancer that has not spread to the lymph nodes.

Nodularity: Increased density of breast tissue, most often due to hormonal changes, which causes the breast to feel lumpy in texture.

Nodules: Small firm tumors.

Noninvasive: Cancer that has not spread into surrounding tissues, such as tissue surrounding the ducts or lobules of the breast. See **ductal carcinoma in situ [DCIS].**

Nonmetastatic: Cancer that has not spread from the primary (original) site to other sites in the body.

Nonpalpable: Cannot be identified by touch.

Nonsurgical biopsy (see also **fine needle aspiration biopsy, core needle aspiration biopsy,** or **stereotactic needle biopsy**): Removal of tissue or fluid by nonsurgical methods, such as with a syringe and needle, for pathological examination.

Nuclear grade: An estimation of a cancerous tumor's potential aggressiveness based on the microscopic examination of the nuclei found within individual cancer cells.

Observation: The person's condition is closely monitored, but treatment does not begin until symptoms appear or change. Also called watchful waiting.

Oncogenes: Genes associated with cancer. *Mutations* in an oncogene can result in altered cell growth and/or behavior.

Oncologist (see **medical oncologist** and **radiation oncologist**): A physician who specializes in cancer treatment.

Oncology: The science dealing with the physical, chemical, and biological properties and features of cancer, including causes, the disease process, and therapies.

Ovaries: Female reproductive organs that produce the eggs required for sexual reproduction. The ovaries are also the major site of estrogen and progesterone production.

Overall survival: Survival that does not take into account whether or not the disease has recurred. Breast cancer survival statistics are often reported in terms of overall survival over a period of time, such as 5 or 10 years.

Paget's disease: Noninvasive breast cancer of the nipple. Paget's disease is often found in association with underlying invasive breast cancers, usually invasive ductal carcinoma.

Palliative therapy: Treatment given to relieve symptoms caused by advanced cancer. Palliative therapy does not alter the course of a disease but improves the quality of life.

Palpable: Identifiable by touch.

Palpation: A procedure using the hands to examine organs such as the breast. A palpable mass is one you can feel with your hands.

Partial mastectomy: A procedure in which part of the breast is conserved by removing only the cancer, some of the breast tissue, the lining over the chest muscles below the tumor, and some of the lymph nodes under the arm.

Partial response: The shrinking, but not complete disappearance, of a tumor in response to therapy. Also called partial remission.

Pathological examination: Evaluation of body tissues, fluids, and organs for disease or injury. Samples are inspected by a pathologist both with the unaided eye and with magnification under a microscope. Special dyes are used to stain or highlight different tissue components.

Pathological staging: A determination of the extent of cancer progression that is based on the results of clinical exam, imaging methods such as mammography, and pathological examination of tissue removed from the breast and/or other sites during biopsy and surgery.

Pathology: The study of disease through the microscopic examination of body tissues and organs. Any tumor suspected of being cancerous must be diagnosed by pathological examination.

Pathology report: The report prepared by the pathologist after examining tissue removed during biopsy or surgery. The pathology report contains information on the tumor's appearance or behavior when viewed both directly and with the aid of a microscope.

Peau d'orange: Term used to describe abnormal dimpling of the breast, similar to the "skin of an orange."

Pectoralis muscles: Muscular tissues attached to the front of the chest wall and extending to the upper arms. These are under the breast.

Permanent section: A technique in which a thin slice of biopsy tissue is mounted on a slide to be examined under a microscope by a pathologist in order to establish a diagnosis.

Phyllodes tumor: Rare, benign, or malignant tumors of the breast.

Plastic surgeon: A surgeon specializing in decreasing disfigurement caused by disease or injury. Breast reconstruction is performed by a plastic surgeon.

Platelet: A cell formed by the bone marrow and circulating in the blood that is necessary for blood clotting.

Ploidy status: The number of chromosome sets contained in a cell. A normal human cell contains 46 chromosomes. Cancerous cells sometimes contain multiple copies of these 46 chromosomes. Also known as DNA index.

Port, life port, port-a-cath: A device surgically implanted under the skin, usually on the chest, that enters a large blood vessel and is used to deliver medication, chemotherapy, and blood products and also is used to obtain blood samples. A port is usually inserted if a person has veins in the arm that are difficult to use for treatment, or if certain types of chemotherapy drugs are to be given.

Positive axillary lymph nodes: Lymph nodes in the area of the armpit (axilla) to which cancer has spread. This is determined by surgically removing some of the lymph nodes and examining them under a microscope to see whether cancer cells are present.

Premalignant: A term used to describe a condition that may be or is likely to become cancer. Also called precancerous.

Primary therapy: The first in a series of measures taken to treat a disease.

Primary tumor: Original site of cancer before spread to secondary tumor sites in the same organ, regional lymph (such as the axillary nodes of the armpit), or distant sites.

Progesterone: Female hormone produced by the ovaries that aids in menstrual cycle regulation. It is key in egg maturation and preparing the uterus for pregnancy. Some breast cancers are activated by progesterone.

Progesterone receptor: A protein in breast cancer and other cells to which progesterone attaches. Progesterone receptors are not present in all breast cancer cells, but a large number of progesterone receptors indicate that progesterone aids the growth of the cancer.

Progesterone receptor status: Determination of whether a tumor's cells contain large or small numbers of progesterone receptors. If the progesterone receptor status is *positive,* the cells contain large numbers of receptors and there is a chance that hormonal therapies will be effective. If the progesterone receptor status is *negative,* the cells do not need the hormone progesterone to grow and usually do not respond to hormonal therapy.

Prognosis: An estimate of the probable disease outcome, based on the distribution of outcomes experienced by a large number of individuals with the same disease characteristics.

Prognostic factors: Elements that contribute to predicting the outcome of a disease. Prognostic factors for breast cancer include axillary lymph node status, tumor size, and the presence of biological markers such as hormone receptors.

Prophylactic bilateral mastectomy: The surgical removal of both breasts before there is evidence of cancer. This procedure is sometimes recommended as a cancer prevention measure in women who are at high risk for developing breast cancer. See **mastectomy.**

Prophylactic contralateral mastectomy: The surgical removal of a healthy breast from the opposite (contralateral) side of the body from a breast diagnosed with breast cancer. This procedure is sometimes recommended as a cancer prevention measure in women who are at high risk for developing another breast cancer. See **mastectomy.**

Prophylaxis: Measures taken for the purpose of preventing a disease.

Prosthesis: Man-made replacement for a removed limb or breast. In the case of breast cancer following mastectomy, a breast form that can be worn inside a mastectomy bra, commonly made of silicone.

Protocol: A schedule of selected drugs and treatment time intervals known to be effective against a certain cancer.

Quadrant: One of four quarters in a three-dimensional object, such as a sphere. The human breast can be divided into the upper left, upper right, lower left, and lower right quadrants.

Quadrantectomy: Surgical removal of a quadrant of the breast and the portion of the lining that covers the chest muscle (but is not the chest muscle itself) that is associated with the removed quadrant. The removed breast quadrant contains the tumor (or tumors) within healthy breast tissue.

Quality of life: The overall enjoyment of life. Many clinical trials measure aspects of a person's sense of well-being and ability to perform various tasks in order to assess the effects that cancer and its treatment have on the person.

Radiation oncologist: A physician who specializes in treating cancer with radiation therapy.

Radiation therapy: Radiation therapy (also called radiotherapy) uses high-energy radiation from X rays, neutrons, and other sources to kill cancer cells and shrink tumors. Radiation may come from a machine outside the body (external-beam radiation therapy) or from materials (radioisotopes) that produce radiation that are placed in or near the tumor or in the area where the cancer cells are found (internal radiation therapy, implant radiation, or brachytherapy). Systemic radiation therapy involves giving a radioactive substance, such as a radiolabeled monoclonal antibody, that circulates throughout the body.

Radiologist: A doctor who specializes in creating and interpreting pictures produced with X rays of areas inside the body.

Radiosensitizers: Drugs that make tumor cells more sensitive to radiation.

Recurrence: The return of cancer at the same site as the original (primary) tumor or in another location, after it had disappeared.

Regimen: A treatment plan that specifies the dosage, the schedule, and the duration of treatment.

Regional: Parts of the body that are located near the site of the primary tumor. For the breast, this includes the skin, chest wall, ribs, lymph nodes inside the chest (internal mammary lymph nodes), and lymph nodes of the armpit (axillary lymph nodes).

Regional control: Removal of all cancerous cells from the region of the body that is near the breast with site-directed treatments such as surgery and radiation therapy. The goal of regional control is to prevent recurrence of the cancer in the skin, chest wall, ribs, and axillary and internal mammary lymph nodes.

Regional involvement: The spread of cancer from its original site to nearby surrounding areas. Regional cancers are confined to one location of the body. Regional involvement in breast cancer could include spread to the lymph nodes or to the chest wall.

Regression: A decrease in the extent or size of cancer.

Relapse: The reappearance of cancer after a disease-free period.

Remission: Complete or partial disappearance of the signs and symptoms of disease in response to treatment. The period during which a disease is under control. A remission, however, is not necessarily a cure.

Retraction: Process of skin pulling in toward breast tissue, often referred to as dimpling.

Risk factors: Anything that increases an individual's chance of getting a disease such as cancer. The risk factors for breast disease are a first-degree relative with breast cancer, a high-fat diet, early menstruation, late menopause, first child after age 30, or no children.

Satellite nodules: Nodules (small firm tumors) located close to a larger primary tumor.

Scans: Pictures of structures inside the body. Scans often used in diagnosing, staging, and monitoring people include liver scans, bone scans, computed tomography (CT) or computed axial tomography (CAT) scans, and magnetic resonance imaging (MRI) scans. In liver scanning and bone scanning, radioactive substances that are injected into the blood stream collect in these organs. A scanner that detects the radiation is used to create pictures. In CT scanning, an X-ray machine linked to a computer is used to produce detailed pictures of organs inside the body. MRI scans use a large magnet connected to a computer to create pictures of areas inside the body

Screening: Checking for disease when there are no symptoms.

Screening mammogram: A breast X ray to detect any possible tumors when there are no findings (such as a lump) during clinical exam to suggest that cancer is present.

Secondary tumor: Cancer that has spread from the organ in which it first appeared to another organ.

Segmental mastectomy: See **partial mastectomy.**

Sentinel lymph node: The first lymph node that cancer is likely to spread to from the primary tumor. Cancer cells may appear first in the sentinel node before spreading to other lymph nodes.

Sentinel lymph node biopsy: Procedure in which a dye and/or radioactive substance is injected near the tumor. This material flows into the sentinel lymph node(s). A surgeon then looks for the dye or uses a scanner to find the sentinel lymph node(s) and removes it (or them) in order to check for the presence of tumor cells.

Side effects: Usually describes situations that occur after treatments. For example, hair loss may be a side effect of chemotherapy; fatigue may be a side effect of radiation therapy.

Skin ulceration: The formation of an open sore on the skin. Skin ulceration on the breast can be a sign of breast cancer.

S phase: Test that is performed to determine how many cells within the tumor are in a stage of division.

S-phase fraction: An indication of the number of tumor cells that are in the process of replicating their DNA in preparation for cell division.

Stage: The extent of a cancer within the body, including whether the disease has spread from the original site to other parts of the body. *Staging* refers to the determination of the extent of cancer.

Stage I breast cancer: Cancer that is no bigger than 2 centimeters (about 1 inch) and has not spread outside the breast.

Stage II breast cancer: Means one of the following: cancer that is no bigger than 2 centimeters but has spread to the lymph nodes in the armpit (the axillary lymph nodes), or cancer that is between 2 and 5 centimeters (from 1 to 2 inches) that may or may not have spread to the lymph nodes in the armpit, or cancer that is bigger than 5 centimeters (larger than 2 inches) but has not spread to the lymph nodes in the armpit.

Stage III breast cancer: Stage III is divided into stages IIIA and IIIB. Stage IIIA breast cancer is defined by either of the following: (1) the cancer is smaller than 5 centimeters and has spread to the lymph nodes in the armpit, which have grown into each other or into other structures and are attached to them, or (2) is larger than 5 centimeters and has spread to the lymph nodes in the armpit. Stage IIIB breast cancer is defined by either of the following: (1) the cancer has spread to tissues near the breast (skin, chest wall, including the ribs and the muscles in the chest), or (2) has spread to lymph nodes inside the chest wall along the breastbone.

Stage IV breast cancer: Cancer has spread to other organs of the body, most often the bones, lungs, liver, or brain. Or the tumor has spread locally to the skin and lymph nodes inside the neck, near the collarbone.

Staging: Doing exams and tests to learn the extent of the cancer within the body, especially whether the disease has spread from the original site to other parts of the body.

Stellate: Appearing on mammography as a star shape because of the irregular growth of cells into surrounding tissue. May be associated with a malignancy or some benign conditions.

Stem cells: The cells from which all blood cells develop.

Stem cell transplantation: A method of replacing immature blood-forming cells that were destroyed by cancer treatment. The stem cells are given to the person after treatment to help the bone marrow recover and continue producing healthy blood cells.

Stereotactic guidance: Use of advanced mammographic imaging technology for precise placement of biopsy needles during fine needle aspiration or core needle biopsy, or "marker" needles and wires during localization procedures performed in preparation for excisional biopsy or lumpectomy.

Stereotactic needle biopsy: Biopsy done while breast is compressed under mammography. A series of pictures locate the lesion, and a radiologist enters information into a computer. The computer calculates information and positions a needle to remove the finding. A needle is inserted into the lump, and a piece of tissue is removed and sent to the lab for analysis. May be referred to as mammotest or core biopsy.

Subcutaneous mastectomy: See **mastectomy.**

Support group: A group of people with a similar disease who meet to discuss how better to cope with their cancer and/or treatment.

Surgical biopsy (see also **excisional biopsy** or **incisional biopsy**): Removal of tissue by traditional surgical methods for pathological examination.

Surgical oncologist: Physician who specializes in cancer surgery.

Surgical margins (also known as resection margins): The region of surrounding normal tissue that is removed along with a tumor during surgery. Resection margins are evaluated by a pathologist to determine whether all of the cancerous tissue was actually removed.

Systemic therapies: Treatments that reach all parts of the body. Systemic therapies for breast cancer include chemotherapy or hormonal therapies given by mouth or intravenous injection. The goal of systemic therapy is to kill all cancer cells in the body, including those that have spread to sites that are distant from the breast.

T cells: One type of white blood cell that attacks virus-infected cells, foreign cells, and cancer cells. They also produce a number of substances that regulate the immune response.

Tamoxifen: Antiestrogen drug in widespread use as an adjuvant hormonal therapy for treatment of breast cancer. Tamoxifen is also under investigation for prevention of breast cancer in women who are at high risk for developing the disease. By binding to the estrogen receptors of breast cancer cells, tamoxifen is able to block the growth-promoting effects of natural estrogen; it is a SERM (selective estrogen receptor modulator).

TNM staging: Classification of the extent of cancer progression based on "T"—the size of the *primary tumor;* "N"—a determination of axillary lymph node spread status; and "M"—the presence or absence of distant metastasis.

Total radical mastectomy: Surgery to remove the breast, chest muscles, and all of the lymph nodes in the armpit. Also called the Halsted radical mastectomy. See **modified radical mastectomy** under **mastectomy** for definition of other type.

Total simple mastectomy: Surgical removal of entire breast, without coremoval of the underlying chest muscles or axillary lymph nodes.

TRAM flap: Method for breast reconstruction in which the abdominal fat tissue is used to form a structure that resembles the breast that was removed during mastectomy.

Tumor (see also **primary tumor** or **secondary tumors**): Abnormal tissue mass formed by uncontrollable cell growth. Tumors are generally classified as malignant (cancerous) or benign (noncancerous). In some cases, the term "precancerous" is used to classify a tumor that has high potential for becoming malignant over time.

Tumor marker: Substances that are sometimes found in an increased amount in the blood, other body fluids, or tissues and that may suggest the presence of some types of cancer. Tumor markers include CA-125 (ovarian cancer), CA-15-3 (breast cancer), CA-25-27, CEA (ovarian, lung, breast, pancreas, and GI tract cancers), and PSA (prostate cancer). Also called biomarkers.

Tumor suppressor gene: Genes that code for proteins that regulate cell growth. Mutations in a tumor suppressor gene can lead to uncontrolled cell growth and the formation of a new or "primary" cancer.

Ultrasound examination: The use of high-frequency sound waves to locate a tumor inside the body. Helps determine if a breast lump is solid tissue or filled with fluids.

Ultrasound guidance: Use of ultrasound imaging technology to direct placement of biopsy needles during fine needle aspiration or core needle biopsy or "marker" needles and wires during localization procedures performed in preparation for excisional biopsy or lumpectomy.

Ultrasound imaging (US): An imaging technology whereby sound waves are reflected off tissues and the echoes are converted into pictures. Microcalcifications cannot be detected by ultrasound.

Ultraviolet radiation: Invisible rays that are part of the energy that comes from the sun. UV radiation can damage the skin and cause melanoma and other types of skin cancer. UV radiation that reaches the earth's surface is made up of two types of rays, called UVA and UVB rays. UVB rays are more likely than UVA rays to cause sunburn, but UVA rays pass deeper into the skin. Scientists have long thought that UVB radiation can cause melanoma and other types of skin cancer. They now think that UVA radiation also may add to skin damage that can lead to skin cancer and cause premature skin aging. For this reason, skin specialists recommend that people use sunscreens that reflect, absorb, and/or scatter both kinds of UV radiation.

Van Nuys classification system: A system developed by investigators in Van Nuys, California, for classifying the risk posed by an individual case of ductal carcinoma in situ. The Van Nuys grade is based on observations made during pathological examination.

Viruses: Submicroscopic organisms that cause infectious disease. In cancer therapy, some viruses may be made into vaccines that help the body build an immune response to and kill tumor cells.

Vital: Necessary to maintain life. Breathing is a vital function.

Watchful waiting: The person's condition is closely monitored, but treatment does not begin until symptoms appear or change. Also called observation.

Wedge resection: See **segmental mastectomy.**

Wire localization: A procedure used to "mark" the boundaries of suspicious sites within the breast with thin, "hook-tailed" wires in preparation for removal by a surgeon during excisional biopsy or lumpectomy. Ultrasound or stereotactic guidance is usually used to identify the sites that need to be marked for surgical excision. Also called needle localization.

X ray: High-energy radiation used in low doses to diagnose diseases and in high doses to treat cancer.

Bibliography

American Cancer Society. *A Breast Cancer Journey: Your Personal Guidebook.* 1st ed. American Cancer Society, 2001.

American Cancer Society. *American Cancer Society's Guide to Complementary and Alternative Cancer Methods.* American Cancer Society, 2000.

Burt, Jeannie, Gwen White, and Judith R. Casley-Smith. *Lymphedema: A Breast Cancer Patient's Guide to Prevention and Healing.* Hunter House, 1999.

Cassileth, B. R. *The Alternative Medicine Handbook: The Complete Reference Guide to Alternative and Complementary Therapies.* Norton, 1998.

Cohen, Deborah A., and Robert M. Gelfand. *Just Get Me Through This: The Practical Guide to Breast Cancer.* Kensington, 2002.

Cranton, Elmer M., M.D., *A Textbook on EDTA Chelation Therapy.* Foreword by Linus Pauling, Ph.D. Hampton Roads, 2001.

Cummings, Stephen, M.D, and Dana Ullman, M.P.H. *Everybody's Guide to Homeopathic Medicines.* Putnam, 1991.

DeGregorio, Michael G., and Valerie J. Wiebe. *Tamoxifen and Breast Cancer.* 2nd ed. Yale University Press, 1999.

Eyre, Harmon, ed., Dianne Partie Lange, and Lois B. Morris. *Informed Decisions: The Complete Book of Cancer Diagnosis, Treatment, and Recovery.* 2nd ed. American Cancer Society, 2001.

Goldberg, Burton W., John Diamond, and W. Lee Cowdin. *The Alternative Medicine Definitive Guide to Cancer.* Future Medicine, 1997.

Harpham, Wendy Schlessel, David M. McPhail (illustrator), and Laura Joffe Numeroff. *The Hope Tree: Kids Talk About Breast Cancer.* Simon and Schuster, 2001.

Kneece, Judy C., R.N., O.C.N. *Helping Your Mate Face Breast Cancer: Tips for Becoming an Effective Support Partner for the One You Love During the Breast Cancer Experience.* 4th ed. EduCare, 2001.

Kneece, Judy C., R.N., O.C.N. *Your Breast Cancer Treatment Handbook*. 3rd ed. EduCare, 1998.

Kneece, Judy C., R.N., O.C.N., and Tricia Brown, eds. *Your Breast Cancer Treatment Handbook: Your Guide to Understanding the Disease, Treatments, Emotions and Recovery from Breast Cancer*. 4th ed. EduCare, 2001.

Labriola, Dan. *Complementary Cancer Therapies: Combining Traditional and Alternative Approaches for the Best Possible Outcome*. Prima, 2000.

Lambert, M. J., and A. E. Bergin. *The Effectiveness of Psychotherapy*. Wiley, 1994.

Lange, Vladimir. *Be a Survivor: Your Guide to Breast Cancer Treatment*. Lange, 1999.

Leung, A. Y., and S. Foster. *Encyclopedia of Common Natural Ingredients Used in Food, Drugs, and Cosmetics*. 2nd ed. Wiley, 1996.

Link, John. *The Breast Cancer Survival Manual: A Step-by-Step Guide for the Woman with Newly Diagnosed Cancer*. Owl Books, 2000.

Love, Susan M., M. D., with Karen Lindsay. *Dr. Susan Love's Breast Book*. 2nd ed. Addison-Wesley, 1995.

Loveland, Foster S. *Herbs for Health*. Interweave Press, 1996.

Lu, Nan, and Ellen Shaplowsky (contributor). *Traditional Chinese Medicine: A Woman's Guide to Healing from Breast Cancer*. Avon Books, 1999.

Nash, Jennie. *The Victoria's Secret Catalog Never Stops Coming: And Other Lessons I Learned from Breast Cancer*. Scribner's, 2001.

Porter, Margit Esser. *Hope Lives! The After Breast Cancer Treatment Survival Handbook*. H.I.C., 2000.

Quillin, Patrick, Ph.D., R.D., C.N.S. *Beating Cancer with Nutrition*. Bookworld Services, 2001.

Rickover, Robert. *Fitness Without Stress: A Guide to the Alexander Technique*. Metamorphous Press, 1988.

Sager, Stephen M. *Restored Harmony: An Evidence-Based Approach for Integrating Traditional Chinese Medicine into Complementary Cancer Care*. Dreaming DragonFly, 2001.

Simone, John. *The LCIS and DCIS Breast Cancer Fact Book*. Three Pyramids, 2002.

Vogel, Carole Garbuny. *Breast Cancer: Questions and Answers for Young Women*. Twenty-First Century Books, 2001.

Weed, Susun S., and Christine Northrup, M.D. *Breast Cancer? Breast Health! The Wise Woman Way*. Ash Tree, 1997.

Weiss, Marisa C., and Ellen Weiss. *Living Beyond Breast Cancer: A Survivor's Guide for When Treatment Ends and the Rest of Your Life Begins*. Times Books, 1998.

Werbach, M. R. *Nutritional Influences on Illness*. 2nd ed. Third Line Press, 1993.

References

INTRODUCTION

American Cancer Society. "Cancer Facts and Figures 2001."

Breast Cancer Action. "The Growth of Patient Advocacy." *Newsletter* 10, February 1992.
National Cancer Institute. "Surveillance Epidemiology and End Results (NCI SEER) program, Cancer Statistics Review (CSR)." Overview; table I-19, 2001.

U.S. General Accounting Office. "1971–1991: Prevention, Treatment and Research." *Breast Cancer,* GAO/PEMD-92-12, 1991.

PART I. 100 QUESTIONS & ANSWERS

CHAPTER 1. BREAST CANCER BASICS

American Cancer Society. "Breast Cancer Questions and Answers." No. 5009.03, April 2001.

American Cancer Society. "For Women Facing Breast Cancer." No. 4652, March 2001.

American Medical Women's Association. "Q & A Hormone Replacement Therapy and Breast Cancer Risk." www.amwa-doc.org. 1999.

Associated Press. "New Treatment Cuts Radiation Time for Breast Cancer Patients." *Dallas Morning News,* February 4, 2002.

Breast Cancer Care. "Fact Sheet: Breast Cancer and Pregnancy." November 2000.

Brenner, Barbara. "Seeing Our Interests Clearly: Follow the Money II." *Breast Cancer Action Newsletter* 52, February/March 1999.

Burstein, H. J., and E. P. Winer. "Primary Care for Survivors of Breast Cancer." *New England Journal of Medicine* 343 (15): 1086, 2000.

Easton, D. F., D. T. Bishop, F. Ford, et al. "Genetic Linkage Analysis in Familial Breast and Ovarian Cancer: Results from 214 Families." *American Journal of Human Genetics,* 52 (4): 678–701, 1993.

Guinee, V. F., H. Olsson, and T. Moller. "Effect of Pregnancy on Prognosis for Young Women with Breast Cancer." *Lancet* 343: 8913, 1994.

John, Lauren. "Male Breast Cancer: An Overshadowed Diagnosis." *Breast Cancer Action Newsletter* 59, May/June 2000.

King, Warren. "Hormone Therapy: High Risk of Breast Cancer." *Seattle Times,* February 13, 2002.

McKie, Robin. "Gene Test Hope on Breast Cancer." *Guardian Unlimited Observer,* February 3, 2002.

NABCO. "Could This Be Breast Cancer?" *NABCO Fact Sheet,* October 2001.

NABCO. "Regional Support Group Database." www.nabco.org/index.php/20.

National Cancer Institute. "Breast Cancer and Pregnancy." (PDQ) Fact Sheet.

National Cancer Institute. "Racial/Ethnic Patterns of Cancer in the United States." No. 96-4104, 1996.

National Cancer Institute. "What You Need to Know About Cancer." No. 00-1566, revised June 2000.

Petrek, J. A., R. Dukoff, and A. Rogat Ko. "Prognosis of Pregnancy-Associated Breast Cancer." *Cancer A* 67 (4): 869–72, 1991.

Rubin, Rita. "To Test, or Not to Test, for Breast Cancer Genes." *USA Today,* January 10, 2002.

Surbone, A., and J. A. Petrek. "Childbearing Issues in Breast Carcinoma." *Cancer* 79: 1271, 1997.

Young, Emma. "Delaying Childbirth Increases Breast Cancer Risk." *NewScientist.com,* February 13, 2002.

Chapter 2. Screening, Mammograms, & Biopsies

American Cancer Society. "Breast Cancer: Early Detection." September 2001.

American Cancer Society. "Guidelines for the Early Detection of Breast Cancer." No. 3304, September 2001.

"BCA's Policy on Mammography." *Breast Cancer Action Newsletter* 66, July/August 2001.

Davis, Devra Lee. "Most Cancer Is Made, Not Born." *San Francisco Chronicle,* August 10, 2000.

Ettinger, Dr. Bruce. "Assessing the Risks." *ABCNews.com,* January 11, 2002.

Evans, Nancy. "Lancet Article Pierces Mammography Balloon." *Breast Cancer Action Newsletter* 34, February 1996.

Hwang, Mi Young. "Know Your Options for Breast Cancer." *JAMA,* February 24, 1999.

John, Lauren. "Thermography: An Alternative to Mammography?" *Breast Cancer Action Newsletter* 60, July/August 2000.

Lyman, Francesca. "Of Mammograms and Millirems." *MSNBC.com,* March 15, 2002.

NABCO. "NABCO Breast Cancer Resource List." 2001/2nd ed.

National Cancer Institute. "The Facts About Breast Cancer and Mammograms." No. 97-3836, September 1997.

"Recommended Breast Cancer Surveillance Guidelines." *Journal of Clinical Oncology* 15: 2149–56, 1997.

Chapter 3. Your Lymph Nodes

Andrews, Alexandra, W. M., Beverley Burns, L.Ac., O.M.D., Sarah Holmes, C.H., Marilyn Miller, C.M.T., L.T., Betty Segal, C.M.T., MaryEllen Sperling, P.T., L.T., and Joanne Thompson. "Helpful Tips for Lymphedema." www.cancerlynx.com

"Cancer and Treatment Information." Memorial Sloan-Kettering Cancer Center, www.mskcc.org.

Erickson, J., et al. "Arm Edema in Breast Cancer Patients." *National Cancer Institute* 93: 96–111, 2001.

Petrek, J. A., and M. C. Hellan. "Incidence of Breast Carcinoma Related Lymphedema." *Cancer* 83: 2776–81, 1998.

Chapter 4. Understanding Your Diagnosis

"Cancer and Treatment Information." Memorial Sloan-Kettering Cancer Center, www.mskcc.org.

"Department of Defense Breast Cancer Decision Guide." www.bcdg.org/diagnosis/staging.html.

Dowlatshahi, K., et al. "Lymph Node Micrometastases from Breast Carcinoma." *Cancer* 80: 1188–97, 1997.

Page, D. L., and R. A. Jensen. "Ductal Carcinoma in Situ of the Breast: Understanding the Misunderstood Stepchild." *Journal of the American Medical Association* 275: 948–49, 1996.

"Prognostic Factors in Breast Cancer." College of American Pathologists Consensus Statement 1999. *Archives of Pathology and Laboratory Medicine* 124: 966–78, 2000.

"Questions to Ask Your Doc After a Breast Cancer Diagnosis." Townsend Letters for Doctors & Patients. *Alternative Medicine Research Foundation Newsletter,* August/September 2001.

Silverstein, M. J., et al. "Can Intraductal Breast Carcinoma Be Excised Completely by Local Excision?" *Cancer* 73: 2985–90, 1994.

Weaver, D. L., et al. "Pathological Analysis of Sentinel and Nonsentinel Lymph Nodes From Breast Carcinoma." *Cancer* 55: 303–306, 1987.

Chapter 6. Mastectomy, Lumpectomy, & Breast Reconstruction

American Cancer Society. "Breast Reconstruction Following Mastectomy." No. 4630, October 2001.

Mock, V., M. Pickett, M. Ropka, E. Lin, K. Stewart, V. Rhodes, R. McDaniel, P. Grimm, S. Krumm, and R. McCorkle. "Fatigue and Quality of Life Outcomes of Exercise During Cancer Treatment." *Cancer Practice* 9 (3): 119–27, 2001.

Moulds, J. E., and C. D. Berg. "Radiation and Breast Reconstruction." *Radiation Oncology Investigation* 6 (2): 8–9, 1998.

National Cancer Institute. "Get Relief From Cancer Pain." No. 94-3735, May 1994.

National Cancer Institute. "Understanding Breast Cancer Treatment: A Guide for Patients." No. 98-4251, September 1998.

National Cancer Institute and Johns Hopkins Oncology Center. "Understanding Cancer Pain." No. 00-4540, September 2000.

Olin, J. J. "Cognitive Function After Systemic Therapy for Breast Cancer." *Onocology* 15: 613–18, 2001.

Pinto, B. M., and N. C. Maruyam. "Exercise in the Rehabilitation of Breast Cancer Survivors." *Psycho-Oncology* 8: 191–206, 1999.

Warner, Jennifer. "Experimental Technique May Reduce the Need for Surgery." *WebMD Medical News,* February 7, 2002.

CHAPTER 7. RADIATION THERAPY

Associated Press. "New Treatment Cuts Radiation Time for Breast Cancer Patients." *Dallas Morning News,* February 4, 2002.

National Cancer Institute. "Radiation Therapy and You." No. 00-2227, October 1998.

CHAPTER 8. CHEMOTHERAPY

Breastcancer.org, "Stress and your Immune System." Live chat, September. 2001.

"The Eleventh Annual European Cancer Conference (ECCO 11)." Proceedings of the American Society of Clinical Oncology, Lisbon, Portugal, October 2001.

Galduroz, J. C., and E. A. Carlini. "The Effects of Long-Term Administration of Guarana on the Cognition of Normal, Elderly Volunteers." *Revista Paulista de Medicina* 114: 1073–78, 1996.

Gerenrich, R. L., and R. W. Hart. "Treatment of Oral Ulcerations with Bacid (Lactobacillus acidophilus)." *Oral Surgery* 30: 196–200, 1970.

James, A. P. R. "Common Dermatologic Disorder." *CIBA Clinical Symposia* 19: 38–64, 1964.

Murray, M. "Common Questions About St. John's Wort Extract." *American Journal of Natural Medicine* 4 (7): 14–19, 1997.

National Cancer Institute. "Chemotherapy and You: A Guide to Self-Help During Cancer Treatment." No. 00-1136, June 1999.

National Cancer Institute. "Eating Hints for Cancer Patients: Before, During and After Treatment." No. 99-2079, July 1997.

National Cancer Institute. "Helping Yourself During Chemotherapy." No. 94-3701, July 1994.

O'Shaugnessy, Joyce, M.D., as told to Sue Rochman. "New Combo: Why Xeloda and Taxotere Extend Survival." *MAMM*, May 2001.

Rauma, A. L., R. Torronsen, O. Hanninen, and H. Mykkanen. "Vitamin B_{12} Status of Long-Term Adherents of a Strict Uncooked Vegan Diet ('Living Food Diet') Is Compromised." *Journal of Nutrition* 125: 2511–15, 1995.

Twombly, Renee. "Early Strike." *MAMM,* May 2001.

CHAPTER 9. HORMONAL THERAPY

Ettinger, Dr. Bruce. "Assessing the Risks." *ABCNews.com,* January 11, 2002.

Evans, Nancy, and Andrea Martin. "Tamoxifen: Rush to Judgment." Breast Cancer Fund, www.breastcancerfund.com.

CHAPTER 10. COMPLEMENTARY & ALTERNATIVE THERAPIES

"Alternative and Complementary Treatments for Cancer: Definitions and Guidelines." *CA-A Cancer Journal for Clinicians* 48 (6): 85–107, 1998.

Bass, Judy. "Stay Strong, Fight Cancer." *Natural Health,* July 2000.

Burzynski, S. "Antineoplastons: The Controversy Continues." (Letter to the editor.) *Journal of the American Medical Association* 269 (4): 475, 1993.

Cassileth, Barrie R., and C. Chapman. "Alternative and Complementary Cancer Therapies." *Cancer* 77: 1026–34, 1996.

"Complementary vs. Alternative Therapy." *Coping,* May/June 2001.

Cooper, Cynthia L. "Complementary Medicines." *MAMM,* April 2000.

Foldeak, S., and G. Dombradi. "Tumor-Growth Inhibiting Substances of Plant Origin. I. Isolation of the Active Principle of Arctium Lappa." *Acta Physical Chemistry* 10: 91–93, 1964.

Green, S. "Antineoplastons: An Unproved Cancer Therapy." *Journal of the American Medical Association* 267 (21): 2924–28, 1992.

Lerner, Michael. "Hedging the Bet Against Cancer." *New York Times Magazine,* October 2, 1994.

Mangles, A. R., et al. "Carotenoid Content of Fruits and Vegetables: An Evaluation of Analytic Data." *Journal of the American Dental Association* 93: 284–96, 1993.

Manner, Harold W. "Facts about Metabolic Therapy." Undated booklet.

Mathews-Roth, M. M. "Systemic Photoprotection." *Dermatol Clinics* 4: 335–39, 1986.

National Cancer Institute. "Questions and Answers About Complementary and Alternative Medicine in Cancer Treatment." *Cancer Fact Sheet,* July 1999.

National Cottonseed Products Association. www.cottonseed.com/

Nauts, Helen Coley. "Immunotherapy of Cancer by Bacterial Vaccines." Paper read at International Symposium on Detection and Prevention of Cancer, New York, April 25–May 1, 1976.

Rosenkrantz, W. "Immunomodulating Drugs in Dermatology," in R. W. Kirk, ed., *Current Veterinary Therapy X* (Philadelphia: Saunders, 1989).

Spiegel, D., et al. "Effective Psychosocial Treatment on Survival of Patients with Metastatic Breast Cancer." *Lancet* 2: 888–91, 1989.

Stein, J. R., and C. A. Borden. "Causative and Beneficial Algae in Human Disease Conditions: Review." *Phycologia* 23: 485–501, 1984.

Studzinski, G. P., and D. C. Moore. "Sunlight—Can it Prevent as Well as Cause Cancer?" *Cancer Ressearch* 55: 4014–22, 1995.

Studzinski, G. P., and D. C. Moore. "Vitamin D and the Retardation of Tumor Progression." In *Nutrition and Cancer.* Boca Raton, Fla.: CRC Press, 1996.

Syracuse Cancer Research Institute. www.scri.ngen.com.

Vickers, Andrew J., and Barrie R. Cassileth. "Unconventional Therapies for Cancer and Cancer-Related Symptoms." *Lancet* 2: 123–29, 2001.

Warburg, O. "On the Origin of Cancer Cells." *Science* 123: 309–14, 1956.

CHAPTER 11. CLINICAL TRIALS

Breastcancer.org. "Background: High-dose Chemo/BMT." October 4, 2001.

Fisher, B., J. P. Constantino, D. L. Wickermen, et al. "Tamoxifen for Prevention of Breast Cancer: Report of the National Surgical Adjuvant Breast and Bowel Project P-1 Study." *Journal of the National Cancer Institute* 90 (18): 1371–88, 1998.

National Cancer Institute. "Fact Sheet: Breast Cancer Prevention Studies." Reviewed December 10, 2001.

National Cancer Institute. "Taking Part in Clinical Trials: What Cancer Patients Need to Know." No. 98-4250, December 1998.

PART II. COMPLEMENTARY CANCER TREATMENT

CHAPTER 14. NUTRITIONAL THERAPY

Arden, G. B., et al. "Monitoring of Patients Taking Canthaxanthin and Carotene: An Electroretinographic and Ophthalmological Survey." *Human Toxicology,* 1989.

Bankhead, Charles. "Mushrooms May Play Role in Breast Cancer Prevention and Treatment." *WebMD Medical News,* December 10, 1999.

Grubbs, C. J., et al. "Effect of Canthaxanthin on Chemically Induced Mammary Carcinogenesis." *Oncology,* 1991.

Prudden, J. F., and J. Allen. "The Clinical Acceleration of Healing with a Cartilage Application." *JAMA,* 1965.

The Breast Center at Johns Hopkins Home Page. "Promoting Good Nutritional Habits for Breast Cancer Patients and Survivors." www.med.jhu.edu/breastcenter/

CHAPTER 15. COMPLEMENTARY & ALTERNATIVE MEDICINE

American Chiropractic Association. www.amerchiro.org/

"Cancell/Entelev (PDQ®)." National Cancer Institute's website, www.cancer.gov, June 2001.

Center for Alternative Medicine Research in Cancer, The University of Texas (Houston) Health Science Center. www.sph.uth.tmc.edu/utcam/default.htm

Greer, S. "Psychological Response to Cancer and Survival." *Psychol Med* 21: 43–49, 1991.

International Taoist Tai Chi Society. www.taoist.org.

Maunsell, E., J. Brisson, and L. Deschenes. "Psychological Distress After Initial Treatment of Breast Cancer," *Cancer* 70: 120–25, 1992.

Nurse Healers-Professional Associates International. www.therapeutic-touch.org/

Quillin, Patrick, Ph.D., R.D., C.N.S. "Antineoplastons." *National Cancer Institute Cancer Facts,* July 13, 2001.

The American Cancer Society. "Questionable Methods of Cancer Management: Cancell/Entelev. *CA—A Cancer Journal for Clinicians,* 1993.

The Burzynski Clinic's Home Page. www.cancermed.com/

The Complete Guide to the Alexander Technique. www.alexandertechnique.com/

The National Association for Holistic Aromatherpy (NAHA). www.naha.org/

Vandeweyer, et al. "Radiation Therapy After Immediate Breast Reconstruction with Implants." *PRS* 106: 56, 2000.

PART III. GUIDE TO BREAST CANCER—RELATED DRUGS

Adriamycin: Pharmacia and Upjohn Company, the maker of Adriamycin, provides additional information at: www.pharmacia.com/products/pharm.asp.

Aredia: Novartis Pharmeceuticals, the maker of Aredia, provides additional information at: www.aredia.net.

Arimidex: Astra Zeneca, the maker of Arimidex, provides additional information at: www.arimidex.com.

Aromasin: Pharmacia and Upjohn Company, the maker of Aromasin, provides additional information at: www.aromasin.com.

Cisplatin: Additional information about Cisplatin is available at: www.cancerbacup.org.uk/info/cisplatin.htm.

Cytoxan: Additional information about Cytoxan is available at: www.tirgan.com/cytoxan.htm.

Decadron: Additional information about Decadron is available at University of California/San Francisco's Carol Franc Buck Breast Care Center's webpage, at: www.ucsfbreastcarecenter.org/chemo_antinausea.html.

Doxil: ALZA Pharmaceuticals, the maker of Doxil, provides additional information at: http://mimi.zoomedia.com/alza/wt/doxil_pi.htm.

Ellence: Pharmacia and Upjohn Company, the maker of Ellence, provides additional information at: www.ellence.com.

Epogen: Amgen, the maker of Epogen, provides additional information at: www.amgen.com/product/AboutEpogen.html.

Evista: Eli Lilly, the maker of Evista, provides additional information at: www.evista.com/index.jsp.

Fareston: CancerBACUP provides more information about Fareston at: www.cancerbacup.org.uk/info/toremifene.htm. Fareston is manufactured by Schering Laboratories/Key Pharmaceuticals.

Femara: Novartis Pharmeceuticals, the maker of Femara, provides additional information at: www.femara.com.

5-FU: Tirgan Oncology Associates, the maker of 5-FU, provides additional information at: www.tirgan.com/5fu.htm.

Herceptin: Genentech, the maker of Herception, provides additional information at: www.herceptin.com.

Kytril: Roche Laboratories, the maker of Kytril, provides additional information at: www.rocheusa.com/products/kytril/pi_tablets.html.

Leukine: Immunex, the maker of Leukine, provides additional information at: www.immunex.com/patient/pa02e1.html.

Megace: Bristol-Myers Squibb, the maker of Megace, provides additional information at: www.bms.com/medicines/data/.

Navelbine: GlaxoSmithKline, the maker of Navelbine, provides additional information at: http://corp.gsk.com/products/prescriptionmedicines.shtml.

Neupogen: Amgen, the maker of Neupogen, provides additional information at: www.neupogen.com.

Nolvadex (tamoxifen): Astra Zeneca, the maker of Nolvadex, provides additional information at: www.tamoxifen.com.

Novantrone: Immunex, the maker of Novantrone, provides additional information at: www.novantrone.com.

Oncovin: Eli Lilly, the maker of Oncovin, provides additional information at: www.lilly.se/produkter/oncovin/allm.html.

Roxicodone: Roxane Laboratories is the maker of Roxicodone. Additional information about Roxicodone can be found at: www.genrx.com/genrxfree/Top_200_2000/Drugs/n1932.HTM.

Taxol: Bristol-Myers Squibb, the maker of Taxol, provides additional information at: www.taxol.com/txbc.html.

Taxotere: Aventis, the maker of Taxotere (docetaxel), provides additional information at: www.taxotere.com.

Wellcovorin: GlaxoSmithKline, the maker of Wellcovorin, provides additional information at: www.glaxowellcome.com/msds/msdslist.htm.

Xeloda: Roche Laboratories, the maker of Xeloda, provides additional information at: www.rocheusa.com/products/xeloda/ppi.html.

Zinecard: For more information on Zinecard, call Pharmacia and Upjohn Company, the makers of Zinecard, at (800) 253-8600.

Zofran: GlaxoSmithKline, the maker of Zofran, provdes additional information at: www.gsk.com/products/zofran_us.htm.

Zoladex: Astra Zeneca, the maker of Zoladex, provides additional information at: www.zoladex.com.

Breast Cancer Word List: "Dictionary of Cancer Terms." National Cancer Institute.

Index

About the Author

Charyn Pfueffer is a professional journalist and columnist living in San Francisco. Her work has appeared in publications such as *Marie Claire, Mademoiselle, Style Magazine, Philadelphia Weekly,* and *The Boston Phoenix.* In addition to her writing, Charyn's work as a Certified Breast Help Specialist and on the Information and Referral Helpline at the Women's Cancer Resource Center has been incredibly fulfilling. Every week, she staffs the phone line and speaks with people affected by cancer. Sometimes they need practical information, like information on drug therapies or how to locate support groups. Other times, callers simply want to talk, cry, and share. It is the calls that require nothing more than listening that are the most moving.

These callers, and the death of Charyn's mother to cancer, are what inspired *Breast Cancer Q & A.* She feels strongly that women should be empowered in all aspects of life, especially when it comes to health issues. The information is out there, but obtaining it can sometimes be frustrating and difficult, particularly when a woman is confused or unaware of her options. She hopes that this book will help ease women's fears during a frightening time and let them know that, ultimately, they are in control of their bodies and lives.

About the Experts

LILLIE SHOCKNEY, R.N., B.S., M.A.S.,
DIRECTOR OF EDUCATION AND OUTREACH AT JOHNS HOPKINS
BREAST CENTER

Lillie Shockney is a registered nurse with a master's degree in administrative science from Johns Hopkins University, where she has been employed since 1983. After her personal experience with breast cancer at the age of 38, Shockney began to contribute additional time to the hospital as a volunteer for the Breast Center. In this role she conducted patient satisfaction surveys, developed quality-of-care measurement methods, and worked with the clinical team to develop ways to improve patient care and services for women diagnosed with breast cancer. In 1997, Shockney joined the Breast Center staff as education and outreach director and webmistress, responsible for quality of care and patient education programs and community outreach.

Shockney has written books and articles on breast cancer, including *Breast Cancer Survivors' Club: A Nurse's Experience.* She is the cofounder of the national nonprofit organization Mothers Supporting Daughters with Breast Cancer and recently became a member of the Advisory Board and Board of Trustees of the National Consortium of Breast Centers, as well as the National Consumer Advisory Council and the Board of the National Women's Health Research Center. She is the recipient of the Outstanding Women of America Award; the National Circle of Life

Award from *Shape* magazine and the National Race for the Cure; the Komen Volunteer Award; Intel's Internet Health Hero Award for the support she provides to patients and families online; and the American Cancer Society's Voice of Hope Award. She has appeared in numerous national magazines and national television programs. In 2000, she was selected as an "Unsung Hero" for breast cancer by Pharmacia and UpJohn's 2001 calendar, and she will be featured in Discovery Health Television's documentary on Hopkins Nursing to air in the fall.

Shockney is a strong advocate of the value of humor as a beneficial form of complementary medicine and speaks on this subject often. Her personal goal is to foster the development and implementation of national quality standards for the diagnosis and treatment of breast cancer in the United States.

BEVERLY BURNS, L.AC., CLINICAL DIRECTOR OF THE CHARLOTTE MAXWELL COMPLEMENTARY CLINIC

Beverly Burns began studying Chinese medicine in 1986 at Quan Yin Healing Arts Center. The following year, after entering the San Francisco College of Acupuncture, she volunteered at the Haight Ashbury Free Acupuncture Clinic. While there, she studied herbal medicine with two herbalists from China, Dr. Jiang Fu Jiang and Dr. Zhu, who specialized in treating cancer and hormonal imbalances.

Since being licensed in 1991, Burns has maintained a private practice in San Francisco and helped establish the Charlotte Maxwell Complementary Clinic, a clinic for low-income women with cancer, for which she now serves as president of the Board of Directors. This clinic is the first acupuncture clinic established as a primary care facility in the state of California. She is the clinical director, evaluating cases of individual clients and training other acupuncturists and herbalists in the treatment of cancer.

In her personal time, Beverly enjoys spending time with her daughter and her partner, traveling, playing team sports, and being involved in community-building with friends and activists.